# A CELEBRATION OF *Sex* FOR NEWLYWEDS

DR. DOUGLAS E. ROSENAU

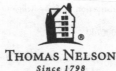

THOMAS NELSON
*Since 1798*

NASHVILLE  DALLAS  MEXICO CITY  RIO DE JANEIRO

Published in Nashville, Tennessee, by Thomas Nelson. Thomas Nelson
is a registered trademark of Thomas Nelson, Inc.

Thomas Nelson, Inc., titles may be purchased in bulk for educational,
business, fund-raising, or sales promotional use. For information,
please e-mail SpecialMarkets@ThomasNelson.com.

Unless otherwise noted, Scripture quotations are from THE NEW KING
JAMES VERSION. Copyright © 1982 by Thomas Nelson, Inc.

Scripture quotations noted NIV are from the HOLY BIBLE:
NEW INTERNATIONAL VERSION®. Copyright © 1973, 1978, 1984
by International Bible Society. Used by permission of Zondervan
Publishing House. All rights reserved.

Illustrations by Alan Tiegreen

**Library of Congress Cataloging-in-Publication Data**

Rosenau, Douglas
    A celebration of sex for newlyweds / Douglas E. Rosenau.
      p. cm.
    ISBN 978-0-7852-8773-5 (tp)
    ISBN 978-0-7852-6523-8 (hc)
    1. Sex in marriage. 2. Sex instruction. 3. Sex—Religious aspects—Christianity. I. Title.
HQ31 .R84253 2002
646.7'8—dc21     2002000740

*Printed in the United States of America*
13 QVS 0 9 8

Two amazing women have so profoundly touched my life. What an awesome example as they were newlyweds in 1942 and 1944 and built passionate marriages over the next fifty years.

They wonderfully model intimacy with their total devotion to Jesus, their gregarious joy in deep friendships, their unselfish nurturing of their families— and in their eighties, they understand and proudly support God's call on their son's life to teach sex.

ERNESTINE HEALAN ROSENAU, MY MOTHER
KATHARINE RHODES BROWN, MY MOTHER-IN-LAW

Two amazing women fought so hard, faithfully reached
for Him. Were an awesome example to other wives
involved in 1912 and 1966 ... and had us writers
... more access to the new church.

They would fully model in time with their
laid devotion to Jesus, their generations with deep
devotion ... their role if the offspring of their families ...
and of their eighties, their one blessed and cheerful
support God will ... darkness ... to each son.

— Ephesians ...
— ... 1 Corinthians ...

# CONTENTS

# INTRODUCTION

*W*elcome to the most important human relationship you will ever build—MARRIAGE! You will feel more deeply and grow wiser in ways you cannot even imagine. You will never be the same again! This book may be one of the most critical you have ever read because it will help you create and enrich what is so unique about marriage, becoming intimate lovers.

Sexuality is that crucial element in marriage that keeps you from simply being roommates over the coming years. In God's design, sex and an intimate marriage can never be separated. He wove sexual fulfillment intricately into the fabric of marital companionship and created the concept of two becoming one flesh in wild, wise, and wonderful ways.

## AVOIDING THE SEXUAL DETOURS

Here's a scary thought: What if you are entering your new sex life in marriage with the wrong map and are going to end up on a very frustrating journey, or even worse—are an accident waiting to happen? There are a lot of myths out there about sex. Perhaps before developing what a great marriage and sex life is all about, some of the sexual detours (false expectations) that have damaged other newlyweds should be mapped out.

*"Sex is natural, and lovemaking will fall into place easily in our marriage." "If we wait till marriage, we will have a great sex life."* Becoming intimate both emotionally and physically takes skills. Time and effort are required to learn to communicate and initiate and disagree. To truly learn your partner's body and how to turn them on does not happen in dating days or on the honeymoon. Your genitals, minds, hormones, and sexual responses are God-given, but you will have to learn to make beautiful music together. Yes, if you wait till marriage you will have fewer wounds and less baggage, but it is still a skill-building process that won't automatically fall into place.

*"Sex is the most important component of a great Christian marriage." "Sex is wild and crazy and the most exciting experience ever."* As an engaged or newlywed couple you may wonder if anything is a close second to sex, but it is not the be-all and end-all in achieving a great marriage. Playing, achieving goals, worshiping, and enjoying intimate relationships are also crucial. But sex, along with your faith and intimate friendship, is indeed indispensable.

Will you re-create the movies and rip each others clothes off and have wild orgasms? Sometimes perhaps. Don't be set up and disappointed like one of my clients. She said she went on her honeymoon expecting sex to be an exciting race car, but felt she came home with a camel. In addition to being unrestrained, lovemaking is also comfortable, a learning process, and warmly connecting. The honeymoon should include a lot of intimate cuddling and learning about each other's bodies, because this is the foundation of wild sex.

*"Great lovers have great technique." "Men/I know all about sex." "Sexual experience correlates with lovemaking skills."* This book stresses being knowledgeable and wisely knowing biology and technique. Sex, bottom line, is not about technique though. The rest of this introduction stresses that great lovemaking is about intimate relating, and Chapter 1 demonstrates that great lovers know how to play, be openly curious, and disciplined. How would men learn all about sex? The locker room is hardly a fount of knowledge. I remember one of my clients who had slept with more than fifty women and yet was one of the most inept lovers I ever counseled. Couples, regardless of experience, must learn each other's unique bodies and responses as they experiment and coach each other.

*"Lovemaking will occur spontaneously and often."* A couple, after being married one month, asked me why they weren't fitting the honeymooner's rabbit syndrome. Then they explained that they had moved out of state, both started new jobs, and were grieving over many losses along with stress of this great adventure. Cut yourselves some slack and be realistic. Even newlyweds need to be aware of optimal times and plan sex into their busy schedules. They will sometimes feel down emotionally and not always be ready to go. This is normal.

*"Sexual mistakes and sins are more difficult to forgive and may haunt for a lifetime."* First Corinthians 6:18 says, "Flee sexual immorality. Every sin that a man does is outside the body, but he who commits sexual immorality, sins against his own body." God did create our bodies to be the home of the

Holy Spirit. Sexual sins are a personal violation of God's home and therefore can have more personal consequences. Masturbating to pornography will create greater fallout in your body and soul than being rude to a friend. This does *not* mean that sexual sins are the worst sins and should create guilt for a lifetime. Our heavenly Father desires to forgive and redeem sexual sins and mistakes just like any other transgressions.

One young lady was dreading sex in marriage and stated she had ruined her wedding night with her past mistakes. I told her that God was not as concerned with her wedding night as He was with the next sixty years. She needed to appropriate His forgiveness and allow Him to redeem her sexuality, as He helped her create a fun intimacy with her new husband.

## GETTING TO THE HEART OF A GREAT SEX LIFE

God has a fantastic formula for your sex life. But great love-making is not for the immature and unskilled. *Only Christlike grown-ups in a committed marriage can make love as the Creator designed!*

### AN INTIMATE MARRIAGE + MATURE LOVERS = A FULFILLING SEX LIFE

Instant sex cannot create instant intimacy. Fulfilling sex flows out of fulfilling intimacy. Developing a fun, trusting companionship takes time and an intimate knowledge of one's partner. In God's design, this companionship precedes fulfilling sexual interaction. Sex is not the most important part of a marriage. A loving companionship and a right relationship with God are the essentials. Even though a great sex life does not ensure a great marriage, a great marital companionship can provide the foundation for fantastic lovemaking.

## BUILDING THE COMPANIONSHIP

The Bible describes the beauty and complexity of the marital companionship that creates the context for lovemaking. This loving, intimate relationship is modeled after the relationship of God with His chosen people. A mature companionship fashions itself after *redemption* in that you die to yourself and let go of any defensiveness and self-centeredness. You create a bonded partnership in which you submit your will for the good of your mate. Your union is based on love and trust and is all about nurturing.

Your trust is well founded because each of you lovingly meets the needs of the other as carefully as you would care for your own body. In this union, you look honestly at your own rough edges and shortcomings and humbly try to change them. You choose to give as precious gifts the things that your mate desires and needs. It is a marvelous atmosphere for fun sexual relating and intimate connecting when this kind of tenderness, trust, genuine empathy, and cooperation abound.

## INCORPORATING REASONABLE BIBLICAL EXPECTATIONS FOR AN INTIMATE MARRIAGE

Most couples enter marriage with a variety of expectations about how it should be. One couple told me that if they could only let go of all their expectations, they would have a happy marriage. I asked them, "Why get married if you don't expect anything from the relationship and your mate?" The task you face is not getting rid of all your expectations but basing them realistically on biblical principles.

Here are seven crucial expectations based on God's guidelines for a fun and intimate marriage. You will find that they actually are the *foundation of great lovemaking,* and their absence will create bumpy detours for even the most promising sex life.

*1. Each of us will become a partner and soul mate offering unconditional love, understanding, and support. We will be best friends:* "The LORD God said, 'It is not good that man should be alone'" (Gen. 2:18).

An important part of cleaving together and becoming one flesh is being intimate companions. You become soul mates and best friends in marriage as you share your souls—your needs, your innermost feelings and desires, your future goals. It is important to have a same-sex best friend who can listen, understand you, and hold you accountable. But your partner should become your very best friend.

*2. We will leave our fathers and mothers and create a new, independent, special family unit. We will learn a healthy independence within our own marriage as each of us creates a life:* "For this reason a man will leave his father and mother and be united to his wife, and the two will become one flesh" (Eph. 5:31 NIV); "Work out your own salvation with fear and trembling; for it is God who works in you both to will and to do for His good pleasure" (Phil. *2:12–13*).

Disentangling yourself financially and emotionally from your parents and family is important. Together you are creating a new partnership and family. You cannot hold on to the need to run back to your parents for constant nurturing. You need to make a definite, symbolic statement that your spouse is your first priority. It does not mean either disrespecting your parents or never leaning on them for support. The act of leaving your parents makes your mate feel special and protected— a priority as you meet your mate's needs. It creates that new and unique partnership.

You must also learn to nurture yourself and work out your own daily walk as you become self-sufficient and confident. If you are insecure and possessive, you can smother your mate. Real love is free of fear and gives breathing room for you and your mate to grow and experience life. You must work on your own happiness as you take responsibility to grow and experience contentment apart from your family and your mate. Be careful not to follow this through to the unhealthy side of being disengaged and too independent. That can be equally destructive.

*3. We will have regular, healthy disagreements. Confrontation around our unmet personal needs will be believed and not dismissed. Either of us will be able to initiate marriage counseling, and the other will be willing to go:* "Correct, rebuke and encourage—with great patience and careful instruction" (2 Tim. 4:2 NIV).

Disappointed expectations, frustrated needs, stored hurt, and retained anger create bitterness and distance and destroy intimacy. You as a couple have to have the courage for healthy conflict and confrontation. Learn conflict-resolution skills, practice forgiveness, and let go of hurt as you resolve differences.

Mates are unique individuals who will be incompatible. The differences can actually enhance a marriage. With good communication skills and the resolution to not let the sun go down on your anger, you will be able to work through these differences. Wise counsel is also a constant source of marital enrichment. It may come from a marriage counselor or mentor to help you learn better communication skills or a financial adviser to help you set up an effective budget; it may come from your pastor to help you work on confession and forgiveness or a sex therapist to help you work on sexual problems. Humbly and courageously work through your disagreements together or as needed with that wise counselor.

*4. We will take regular vacations and honeymoons throughout our marriage as we mend and enhance our intimacy:* "To everything there is a season, / A time for every purpose under heaven: / A time to break down and a time to build up" (Eccles. 3:1, 3).

There should be some special time set aside for a honeymoon and more concentrated, focused time in that first year together. It is a time of adjusting and getting to know each other. The marital plague of today is being overinvolved and too busy. Give yourself permission to budget time and money for your partnership. Busy couples cannot maintain the level of intimacy they desire without regular time away on date nights, weekends away, and longer vacations.

5. *We will use credit carefully as we become wise stewards of our finances:* "Owe no one anything except to love one another" (Rom. 13:8).

A great sex life is closely dependent on staying out of debt and learning to handle finances wisely. It makes sense that any stressors in a marriage will weaken intimacy and the desire to make love. Learn to be self-disciplined in this area of your life. Mutually agree on the partner in your marriage who has the greatest organization and discipline, and then delegate her or him to run the checkbook. Spend less than you make. Financial counselors especially advise against spending excessive money on depreciating items such as cars, clothes, or furniture. Not borrowing money certainly means not using credit cards as you create sound spending and budget habits. Effective stewardship of your finances will indeed enhance your sex life.

6. *We will have regular, satisfying sexual interaction:* "The husband should fulfill his marital duty to his wife, and likewise the wife to her husband. The wife's body does not belong to her alone but also to her husband. In the same way, the husband's body does not belong to him alone but also to his wife. Do not deprive each other" (1 Cor. 7:3–5 NIV).

A reasonable expectation in a good marriage is frequent and mutually fulfilling sexual activity. Couples often ask, "What is the average frequency of making love?" This will truly vary from couple to couple, and some weeks it will be easier to find the time and energy. But, at least twice a week seems a good rule of thumb. Each partner can expect help from the other to experience personal sexual satisfaction. It is realistic to desire and work toward intimacy-enhancing sexual companionship that grows over the years—sexual communication that is much more than just intercourse or orgasm.

It will require an investment by both mates to ensure time, provide variety, and avoid routine. It may also require some counseling to break through any difficulty: an inability of the wife to experience an orgasm, an inability of the husband to last long enough, a wife's or husband's lack of desire, sexual addictions or compulsions, or other problems. Don't put it off; these problems usually won't go away but will get worse. Get help if you are not enjoying regular, satisfying sexual interaction.

*7. We will enjoy a growing spiritual life together with prayer and Bible study:* "Let the word of Christ dwell in you richly . . . Continue earnestly in prayer" (Col. 3:16; 4:2).

Bible study and prayer enhance intimacy and allow you to become more Christlike. God is the author of intimacy, and keeping centered in Him is the beginning of wisdom and an intimate marriage. If you are humble and open, He will shine His truth and love into your life and relationships.

One husband was excited about a discovery he had made: Christians have the ability to be the best lovers in the world. He had read Galatians 5:22–23: "But the fruit of the Spirit is love, joy, peace, longsuffering, kindness, goodness, faithfulness, gentleness, self-control." What a list of traits as a foundation for a great marriage and sex life! If you are filled with God's Spirit and living out these virtues, you will never be surpassed as a marital partner or sexual lover!

# 1

# THE WORLD'S GREATEST LOVER

*F*antastic lovemaking is based on being a fantastic person. Christlike traits and attitudes are what count. True sexiness and a tremendous sex life depend not only on a great marriage but also on being a mature, sexy person.

## AN INTIMATE MARRIAGE + MATURE LOVERS =
## A FULFILLING SEX LIFE

So you want to be the world's greatest lover? Build into your mind and heart the following character traits possessed by all great lovers. These guidelines, gleaned from the Bible, will lead to great sex. Their effective use will show you how to truly arouse your mate's desire. Success is practically guaranteed, but it will take some real prioritizing and practice to incorporate them into your life.

## PLAYFULNESS

Playfulness is perhaps best described by the words *excitement, curiosity, laughter, eagerness*, and *spontaneity*. Playfulness is the ability to be unpretentious and unashamed as you demand things with enthusiasm and childlikeness. In your

1

child ego state, your needs are important and fun and you expect pleasure.

You cannot *work* at creating better lovemaking—you and your mate have to *play* at it. This character trait can be practiced in other areas of your life and the lessons brought back into your sex life. Get silly; anticipate an event for a week or more; risk a new behavior; laugh until you have tears in your eyes or roll on the floor; tickle and chase each other around the whole house; get wide-eyed with awe and wonder about something. You are becoming a great lover.

## LOVE

The Bible says you are to love your neighbor or your mate just as you love yourself. Fun sex depends on a husband and wife who have learned to love themselves. This means you take care of your health and exercise your body to keep it in shape. You also need to work through to accepting and enjoying the body God gave you. Self-acceptance, self-esteem, and a good body image are healthy parts of sexiness and Christian self-love. Think of how difficult it is to sexually focus on your mate when you are embarrassed, inhibited, or self-conscious.

Another important part of love is respecting and unconditionally accepting your mate. If you want to find and focus on flaws, you will put a damper on your partner's sexiness and the whole lovemaking process. You reap the benefit (or destructiveness if you stay obsessive) of nurturing and helping your lover revel in sexual appeal. Every time you affirm some particular aspect of masculinity or femininity that you admire and enjoy, you lovingly increase your mate's sex appeal.

Unconditional love and acceptance and affirmation set the temperature for some fantastic sex.

This may actually need to be emphasized as a separate virtue, but a loving person is a humble, *forgiving* person. If you really desire a fantastic love life, let go of the mistakes your mate makes and heal the disappointed expectations. Cut each other slack and gently, graciously acknowledge that you are both just human. Learn to laugh over shortcomings and revel in the intimacy that comes after working a problem through to an intimate forgiveness.

Love creates trust so you can try new behaviors and risk appearing silly. Love produces warm excitement and fun companionship. Love helps you to remember and desire to meet your mate's needs. Learn to be a lover! The best sex is long-term, and love is the oil that keeps this type of lovemaking running smoothly.

## KNOWLEDGE

There are three parts of being a wise and knowledgeable lover. *First,* become a student of your mate. An integral aspect of true consideration is constantly trying to know and understand your partner better. Lovemaking should be knowing what your mate enjoys and needs. This knowledge takes time, curiosity, a good memory, and the willingness to be a student. Get a Ph.D. in your mate.

*Second,* be an informed and sexy lover by knowing your own body and sexual responses. You are the teacher of your mate. Do you know what turns you on and increases your desire? It will be difficult teaching your erotic needs to your partner if you are not aware of them. Tune in to your sexuality, and keep expanding your repertoire of sensual delights. Learn to become more easily and strongly orgasmic.

*Third,* develop a technical knowledge of sexuality. Sexual technique is not the be-all and end-all of a great sexual relationship, but its importance cannot be denied. Several chapters of this book are about technique. The couple with their act together sexually know how to create ambience and be uninhibitedly sensual and playful. They understand various positions of intercourse, and they have built a comfortable, exciting repertoire of sexual moves.

## HONESTY

In making love, dishonesty destroys trust, allows boredom, and creates confusion and hostility. Great sex is based on mature lovers who can be honest with themselves and their mates. They are self-aware and can *assertively communicate.*

Many couples find it uncomfortable to initiate sexual conversations and openly discuss individual needs and desires. The wife may be upset because her husband gets defensive or pouts if she openly refuses sex or makes a small suggestion. The husband may be angry because his wife turns him down after he plays the romantic rituals like taking a quick shower or rubbing her back. These are times for great air-clearing, honest discussions, and confrontation as the couple openly express feelings and needs.

## CREATIVE ROMANCE

Sexy lovers take the time to develop the sensual, romantic parts of their minds and personalities. Mates can be surprised how talented and creative they are in planning sexy surprises for each other. This may include gifts, foot and leg massages, verbal demonstrativeness, mutual showers, or dinners with candlelight and soft glances. Of course, romantic lovemaking doesn't always involve completely new techniques and experiences. There are certain positions, ways of caressing, places, rhythms, restaurants, moods, and vocabulary that remain enjoyable favorites.

Sexiness comes from your imaginative creativity and romantic inspirations—and the discipline (time and energy) to carry them out. You want to be a great, sexy lover? Become a creative romantic who invests time and energy wisely.

## DISCIPLINE

Discipline may seem an odd character trait to include for a lover, and the opposite of spontaneity, playfulness, and creativity. The truth of the matter is that an undisciplined lifestyle will end up with very infrequent sex. Perhaps you think that discipline would completely destroy the fun and spontaneity of sex and put pressure on you. But if you don't plan sex into your busy schedules and find those optimal times, you will never make love! The ambience, activity, place, timing, and technique are up to your romantic creativity. Just keep a time sacredly (one definition of *sacred* is: "dedicated to a special purpose") reserved for sex.

## A BIBLICAL CELEBRATION

God wants you to prosper as a lover. Immerse yourself in playfulness, love, knowledge, honesty, creative romance, and discipline. In addition, here is some further godly wisdom that can help ensure that your celebration of sex flourishes.

*Enjoy the incompatibility of gender differences.* "So God created man in His own image; . . . male and female He created them" (Gen. 1:27). It is fascinating how often in marriage counseling that gender differences come up. Ways in which the genders vary sexually will be developed more in Chapters 8 and 9. From dating days through the honeymoon and into years of marriage, you will be continually amazed how different you are.

Men need to be made significant and their egos stroked, while women need to feel secure and special. Men tend to be more one-track, whereas women can multitask more easily. Men have a narrower band of emotions, and wives self-disclose and express feelings more adeptly. Women overall desire emotional connection and physical affection as a way to connect their souls and then sex can blossom. Paying attention with phone calls and doing the vacuuming can increase female sexual desire. Men connect their feelings and souls through sexual activity. Being a student of the opposite sex and understanding how your spouse is similar and different from these stereotypes are crucial as you develop into a great lover.

*View sex as a means to an end and never an end in itself.* "Drink water from your own cistern, and running water from your own well . . . Let your fountain be blessed, and rejoice with the wife of your youth. As a loving deer and a graceful doe, let her breasts satisfy you at all times; and always be enraptured with her love" (Prov. 5:15, 18–19). Sex should never be just a physical rush, but a tender, passionate connection. Without the playful, loving companionship, sex becomes another buzz that loses its perspective and has increasingly diminishing returns. Whether it is alcohol, cocaine, or sex, when we artificially try to create highs, we need bigger and better buzzes to keep maintaining the rush. Making love is different. This intense drink of cold water from your endlessly varied supply can be enjoyed throughout the years of your marriage and remain exciting. Why? Because sex is a relationship, not just a physical high.

*Understand that enjoying sexuality and connecting with your mate are gifts each brings to the other willingly—not by demands or coercion.* Please don't use God's loving guidelines as weapons on each other. First Corinthians 7:3, 5 tells about the importance of keeping sexually united in marriage: "Let the husband render to his wife the affection due her, and likewise also the wife to her husband . . . Do not deprive one another except with consent for a time . . . and come together again so that Satan does not tempt you because of your lack of self-control." Some husbands and wives club their mates with this passage and say things like, "If you don't have sex with me tonight, you are sinning." The real sin is theirs because they usually have never taken the time, lovingkindness, and energy to make changes needed to appeal to their mate romantically. Making love is about giving—not demanding.

On the other hand, if you are not giving you may need to push yourself to discover what is wrong and overcome your barriers. This passage does emphasize that mates should be in a place to enjoy sex as a mutual celebration.

*Emphasize feelings in your lovemaking.* There is no replacement for what God intended sex to do for intimate marriages. It is the framework for expressing many powerful and exciting emotions such as joy, love, trust, and playfulness. Making love also helps dissipate and defuse negative emotions and behaviors such as hostility, nit-picking, and defensive distancing. Above all, learn to be passionate. Communicate feelings with your eyes and your hands and your mouth. Let the child ego state reign and squeal with delight and silliness. Laugh lightheartedly as well as intensely groan with pleasure.

*Maximize your imagination.* The Bible talks much about our minds and imaginations with the potential for good or evil. Your mind is the most important sexual organ with its ability to create erotic imagery, fantasies, and feelings. Godly fantasy is focused on your mate and maintains a fun, playful attitude. Your mental imagery should never replace or diminish your mate. It should enhance lovemaking as you store up great memories to replay, brainstorm on creative and arousing activities, and playfully stir up romance.

*Practice righteous selfishness.* As individuals, we are responsible for developing our own sexuality and celebrating love. We need to understand our own sexual needs and assertively fulfill them. God encourages autonomy and personal responsibility for our lives, our bodies, and our sexuality.

Orgasms are an excellent example of healthy sexual selfishness. Your mate does not experience your orgasm. You focus on your sexual feelings and allow them to build to a climax. This is an intensely personal pleasure within your mind and body. You selfishly let your mind enjoy the intensity of your excitement. Your partner is aroused by your personal excitement and intense experiencing of erotic release. This selfishness creates a mutual intimacy that is fun and bonding.

Attention to self and passionately expressing your own pleasure is indeed a great turn-on to you and your mate.

*Bring God's love and values into your marriage and lovemaking.* There have been many different interpretations about what is permissible for a Christian as you browse among the lilies and taste the choice fruits of your marital sexual garden. An example of this would be the different views about oral sex. Though the Song of Solomon seems to imply oral sex, the Christian community has often been skeptical of this behavior, sometimes for unworthy reasons such as viewing the genital area as "dirty" or "too private" or that intercourse is the only natural sexual activity.

When the Bible does not directly deal with a behavior like oral sex or masturbation, we turn to other scriptural values to help govern our sexual behaviors. In light of other injunctions, oral sex can be enjoyed as one of many ways to make love, though some couples may choose not to engage in this expression of love. Whether oral sex, using a vibrator, or trying new positions, we are called to be lovingly considerate and wise. Never should we do anything that violates our mate's sensibilities or offends our mate sexually. (Note: Mates wonder about vibrators in sex. For some women it helps them become more easily orgasmic and for other couples can be a playful prop. The caution would be in producing sensations that the husband cannot duplicate or allowing any prop to detract from a playful, intimate, and varied lovemaking.)

*Become naked and unashamed.* We as lovers are to entrust our private parts only to our mates, for indeed "my own vineyard is mine to give" (Song 8:12 NIV), and we should learn to have no shame or inhibitions with the genital area. Making love is an intimate connecting and a breaking down of walls so that "my lover is mine and I am his [hers]." You are willingly naked and vulnerable. Lovers are able to experience freedom and abandonment together based on love, trust, and commitment. It is a totally unique companionship and so exciting to be naked and not ashamed as you celebrate marriage.

### TIME OUT . . .

*Play.* Buy toys that you and your mate can enjoy together, such as water pistols, jump ropes, rub-on tattoos, or building blocks.

*Love.* Stand nude in front of a full-length mirror. Now observe yourself and resist making any judgments. After observing a few minutes, start with your hair and proceed down to your feet, accepting and describing every one of your body parts with no negative judgments.

*Become knowledgeable.* Take a minute to do a quick personal inventory. Which areas of your sex life can benefit from greater knowledge?

*Be honest.* As you develop into a great lover, periodically ask yourself these questions: Have I developed any dishonest sexual games? Do I sulk or pout rather than talk through my needs? When my needs are satisfied, do I stop or press through to also satisfying my mate's needs? In honesty, work through these issues with your mate.

*Be romantic.* How would you define *romantic*? Make a brief list of behaviors that you consider romantic and do one or two this week.

*Be disciplined.* Put your heads together and plan when and how often you are going to make love each week.

# 2

# YOUR EROGENOUS ZONES

*W*hat an erotic concept, erogenous zones. They are parts of the body that have a concentration of sensory nerve endings, which can be stimulated to cause sexual arousal. Why do we experience a sexual touch or an erotic sight and begin to get an erection or vaginal lubrication? Because God has designed our bodies so that our hormones, nerve endings, and minds naturally create sexual arousal. All you have to do is simply relax and tune in to your God-given erogenous zones, responses, and that most important sexual organ, your mind and imagination.

## HORMONES AND THE AUTONOMIC NERVOUS SYSTEM

Hormones and the nervous system operate in a cooperative process—the hormones activate the process in our bodies and bloodstream, and then our nerves relay sexual information from our senses (eyes, fingertips) to our brains, and back to our genitals to create physical arousal.

Without getting too technical, the autonomic, or involuntary, nervous system is involved in the sexual arousal cycle. It has two branches called the *sympathetic* (SNS) and the *parasympathetic* (PNS). The PNS and the SNS operate in opposite manners. The parasympathetic is operative when we are relaxed, and it has a creative, building effect on the body. The sympathetic springs into action when we are intensely aroused to trigger orgasm, or when we are threatened to shut down the PNS. Both arousal and orgasm are involuntary, reflexive actions. You simply have to relax and enjoy the stimulation of each other.

Because of a conservative Christian background, natural shyness, or discomfort with their bodies, some mates cannot comfortably access their sexuality. This is an important task of the honeymoon and the first year. The hormones and nervous system are obviously in place, and they probably experience some aspects of arousal, but the parasympathetic system needs to be turned loose as the person tunes in to and relaxes with pleasurable sexual feelings. Mates have many fun, sexual discoveries to make in their erogenous zones as they increase their sexual awareness and sensuality.

## EROGENOUS ZONES

Sensuality and sensitivity to touch have to be developed and connected to your sexual lovemaking. Overall, our erogenous zones are more alike than different, whether we are male or female, experienced or inexperienced, overweight or underweight, active or inactive. But some individuals will experience more sensitivity and arousal from certain erogenous points than from others. That is why you must continually be a student of your mate and learn every inch of the body—remembering what is arousing but not locking into boring patterns of stimulation.

The erogenous areas can be divided into three levels according to their sensitivity in producing sexual arousal:

*Level Three.* The entire body with its skin and nerve endings. You may be exclaiming, "Why is the whole skin area considered erogenous? When I rub my arm, I don't get turned on." Actually, the skin is the most extensive area of sensuality, and the whole body enjoys being massaged.

Massage and caress your lover's arms, shoulders, outer ears and earlobes, scalp, upper chest, buttocks, and calves. They may not have the concentration of sensory nerve endings as other parts of the body, but they are still very sensual. They can contribute to a delightfully connecting experience.

*Level Two.* The parts of the body, excluding genitals and nipples, with greater nerve endings and blood supply. These areas supply great stimulation during foreplay. If you desire to be a great lover, become familiar with these spots on your partner's body.

Take fingertips or mouth and tongue and stimulate the delightfully sensory nerve endings of Level Two erogenous zones. Experience the pleasurable feelings of (1) the back of the knees, (2) the inner thighs, (3) the armpits and breast area, (4) the abdomen area and the navel, (5) the small of the back and buttocks, (6) the neck from back to front, (7) the palms of the hands and bottoms of the feet, (8) the face, especially the eyelids and eyebrows, (9) the edges of the nose over the sinus cavities, (10) the temples, (11) and the mouth and

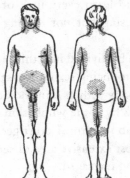

Figure 2.1
Erogenous zones

tongue. Allow these gentle touches, nibbles, and licks to be a sensual treat and to become arousing sexually too.

*Level One.* The most sensitive and sexually stimulating erogenous zones are the nipples and the genitals. The genitals most directly stimulate sexual arousal. The nipples are a favorite spot of both men and women for stimulating sexual excitement. The nerve endings are especially sensitive and connected to sexual arousal. Remember! Level One erogenous zones should not be the immediate focus of loveplay. Tease, caress, and play in the other levels first.

## THE MALE GENITALS

The male genitals are more visible to the eye and familiar to the man because, unlike the woman, he handles his penis every time he urinates. Many men, though, have never taken the time to truly examine their genital area.

*The penis.* The penis is composed of three columns of spongy

*Figure 2.2*
The internal and external male organs

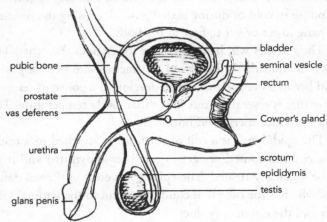

tissue with the urethra running through the bottom column (corpus spongiosum). These spongy tissues fill with blood in a type of hydraulic system that creates the erection. The whole penis is an intricate network of blood vessels and nerves, with the head or glans of the penis being especially sensitive. The skin of the penis is loosely attached to allow for more easy stimulation. Penises can vary in the angle of erection, shape of the head of the penis, width, length, and color. This has nothing to do with the ability to give and receive pleasure. The importance of penis size in making love is indeed a myth. When flaccid, the size of the penis will vary greatly; when erect, the size for most men is about six inches, plus or minus an inch and a half. The outer third of the vagina is the most sensitive, and it would take a penis only three inches or less in length to create great pleasure.

*The scrotum and testes.* The scrotum is a sac of skin enclosing the testes. Under the skin is a muscle that can contract in response to cold or during sexual arousal, causing the scrotum to hang lower or get tighter to the body.

The testicles will hang with one lower than the other. The testes are outside the body and contract toward the body with cold because the sperm need to develop in a constant temperature that is several degrees lower than body temperature. The testes produce sperm and hormones.

The epididymis is a coil of small tubes attached to a testis. The coil can sometimes get infected (epididymitis) and need to be medically treated. The epididymis ends in the vas deferens, which is the tube that conducts sperm to the seminal vesicles and the ejaculatory duct.

*The seminal vesicles, bladder, prostate, and urethra.* As you trace the vas deferens, it becomes a complex valve system with the seminal vesicles, the bladder, and the urethra, which passes through the prostate. The vas deferens brings sperm to the seminal vesicles that form the ejaculatory duct. This duct runs through and joins the urethra in the prostate. The prostate is about the size of a chestnut and, along with the seminal vesicles, produces fluid that forms part of the semen.

## THE MALE GENITAL EROGENOUS ZONES

*Nipples.* The male's nipples are sensitive to touch and create pleasurable feelings when stimulated orally or manually, often becoming hard just like the female's.

*Penis.* The wife will often need her husband to demonstrate the strokes he appreciates most on his penis. Manual stimulation is usually more firm, with the whole hand encircling the organ, and often more rapid, especially when approaching orgasm, than she might expect. The underside of the penis is often very sensitive and responds well to fingertip stroking. The greatest concentration of nerve endings is in the head of the penis. Oral stimulation, the hand well-lubricated, or the vagina create arousal. Again, it will need to be firm stimulation, or it will not be felt or appreciated as much. A wife can place her hand over her husband's hand and learn the strokes and rhythms he enjoys the most. He can also coach on the positions of intercourse that are more stimulating.

*Scrotum and testicles.* The testicles are sensitive to being hit but can be touched quite firmly if done gently. These very erotic parts of a man's body create sensations with caressing or lightly tugging on the scrotal sac.

*Perineum.* This is the area between the scrotum and the anus. It is over the prostate gland as well as being at the base of the penis. It can be quite exciting to rub this area with moderate firmness—especially if done in conjunction with manually stroking the penis with the other hand. Experiment and discover what feels most exciting and pleasurable in loveplay.

## THE FEMALE GENITALS

The vulva comprises the external genitals of the female. The vulva varies greatly in shape and size of outer and inner lips and density of pubic hair from woman to woman. The vulva begins in front with the mons pubis covered with pubic hair and extends down to the perineum above the anus. On either side are the outer labia and inner labia with the clitoris, followed by the urethral opening and the vagina.

*The mons pubis and labia majora.* The pubic mound (mons pubis) is soft tissue over the pelvic bones. It is covered with hair and acts as a cushion during the thrusting of intercourse. The outer lips (labia majora) start down at the anus and extend up to meet at the mons. They are soft folds of tissue that, with the hair on them, protect the inner organs and are often all that are visible as they come together over the inner lips. During sexual arousal, the outer lips become engorged with blood and become flatter.

*The clitoris hood and labia minora.* The inner lips (labia minora) are hairless and start at the vaginal opening and extend upward to meet at the clitoral hood. If the hood is pulled back, the external part of the clitoris can be seen, like a small pea in size. The inner lips vary greatly in size and shape among females. With some women they are larger and extend

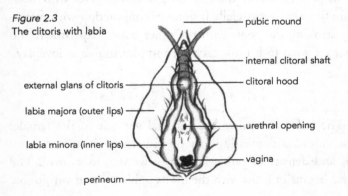

*Figure 2.3*
The clitoris with labia

pubic mound

internal clitoral shaft

external glans of clitoris

clitoral hood

labia majora (outer lips)

urethral opening

labia minora (inner lips)

vagina

perineum

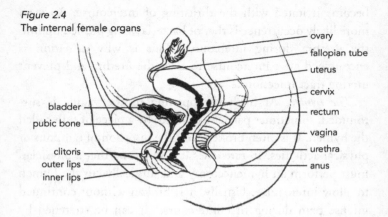

*Figure 2.4*
The internal female organs

ovary
fallopian tube
uterus
cervix
rectum
vagina
urethra
anus

bladder
pubic bone
clitoris
outer lips
inner lips

outside the outer lips. There is no perfect size, but each unique shape will become intensely erotic to the woman's husband. The inner labia become engorged during sexual arousal and change color and increase in thickness. They create a chute that the penis travels down for penetration of the vagina.

*The clitoris and shaft.* The clitoris is homologous to the penis and contains the most sensitivity. It is given to the female solely for sexual pleasure, and stimulating it is the key to tension buildup and climax. During sexual arousal, the clitoris doubles in size and becomes hard like the penis. The clitoral shaft (shaded darker in Figure 2.3) is primarily beneath the surface of the skin under the clitoral hood. When erect it can be felt like rubbing over an electrical wire under a light blanket.

*The urethral opening.* The urethral opening is between the clitoris and vaginal opening but is small and sometimes difficult to detect. The urethra has nothing to do with sexual arousal but is located near the wall of the vagina and can become irritated with the thrusting of intercourse. An even more likely occurrence is that of bacteria being pushed up into the urethra during intercourse. This is why urination is encouraged after intercourse to clear the urethra and prevent uterine tract infections.

*The hymen.* At birth the opening to the vagina is surrounded, sometimes partially covered, by a piece of skin called the hymen. It is often broken with the insertion of tampons or physical activities. In rare cases it is so strong that a physician must perform an hymenectomy and surgically cut the hymen to allow intercourse. Usually, it is broken without continued intense pain during first intercourse. It can be stretched by inserting the thumb or two fingers and gently pushing or pulling before first intercourse.

*The vagina.* The vagina is a shaft or tube of tissue with the sides touching. It is around three inches in length; it is muscular and expands so that it can accommodate any size of penis, especially with arousal. With arousal, the outer third of the vagina swells and creates the orgasmic platform, and the inner part balloons. After arousal, the greater penile stimulation will occur at the mouth, or outer third, of the vagina.

The cervix is at the upper end of the vagina and opens into the uterus. It can be sensitive to the hard thrusting of intercourse, but there are front and rear fornices on either side of the cervix. The rear fornix takes most of the hard thrusts of vigorous intercourse and is designed to collect the semen and hold it near the cervix to increase the likelihood of insemination. The vagina has folds of skin and sweats out lubrication when sexually aroused to allow intercourse. The vagina is delicately balanced with bacteria and acidic fluids to slow down bacterial growth. Be cautious with douches or placing a finger that has been near the bacteria of the anus within the vagina and upsetting the balance.

## THE FEMALE GENITAL EROGENOUS ZONES

*The breasts and nipples.* The breasts and nipples are very exciting to both husband and wife. The husband enjoys the unique femininity of his wife's breasts and sees the nipples becoming erect as an obvious sign of sexual arousal. He needs to remember that his wife will not usually appreciate a direct attack on the nipples or genital area. A woman more often appreciates an indirect, teasing approach. It is also wise to understand that a woman more than a man will vary in what feels stimulating or irritating from one lovemaking session to another. Nipples, for instance, can be affected by hormonal fluctuations. Always be creative as you caress, nibble, lightly touch, or stroke more firmly. Vary the direction and type of stroking as you invite and remember suggestions.

*The labia.* The outer and inner lips have many nerve endings and create sexual excitement. Again, vary the touch as you start with the outer lips and mons. Place the whole hand over the genital area; run a finger from bottom to top of the outer labia; lightly rub the labia together over the clitoral area. Allow sexual tension to build. The penis is a marvelous wand for creating pleasure, especially the soft head. Use it to gently stimulate the inner labia and the clitoris. Let the tension begin to build before active stimulation of the clitoris.

*The clitoris.* The wife will have to discover the strokes and places that she prefers for clitoral stimulation and teach her partner. She may have to slowly sensitize herself to experiencing the fun sensations her clitoris can provide. She can suggest techniques for her husband to use that are helpful for arousing her and creating the rhythm that she needs. Direct stimulation, unless highly aroused, can often be too intense; instead you can rub on the side of the clitoral hood or use the mouth more gently.

*The vagina.* The outer third of the vagina is the most sensitive. This sensitivity should be kept in mind with either manual or penile stimulation. Quick, shallow thrusts, as well as slow, sensual, longer motions, can be very arousing. Often there is greater sensation at twelve o'clock (toward the clitoris) and six o'clock (toward the anus) within the vagina. Positions that stimulate these areas create exciting sensations.

*The perineum and areas adjacent to the vulva.* The perineum, or tissue between the anus and vagina, is sensitive to touch. Any skin or tissues immediately surrounding the vulva are categorized as Level Two erogenous zones and would include areas such as the inner thighs and stomach. Though not the direct genital area, they are very sensitive to caresses, licking, and teasing strokes— almost becoming an extension of the vulva. Remain creative and varied as you enjoy Level One and Level Two erogenous zones.

## SENSUAL EROTIC PAIRING

Sensual erotic pairing or conditioning takes place in your mind as you stimulate the erogenous zones or sensually (touch, sight, smell) notice them and associate (pair) these experiences with hormones and sexual arousal. As you become more aroused, more hormones are released, and you can continue to pair various touches and visual experiences so that they become sexually arousing to you—like kissing or observing your mate's genitals. This is the beauty of a long-term intimate companionship. The pairing/conditioning never ceases, and stored in your mind are many sexually arousing symbols that you can draw on to create or enhance sexual arousal. Stimulating the erogenous zones can continually become charged with sensual and erotic pleasure over a lifetime of lovemaking.

Relax, explore, caress, pair, discover, stroke, expand, touch, and sensuously feel as you fully enjoy God's wonderful gift of sexual pleasure.

### TIME OUT . . .

Let the husband get into a comfortable position lying on his back. The wife is going to gently and carefully explore and touch the genital area from perineum to the tip of the penis. Observe the penis both flaccid and erect. Let him tell her what feels especially sensitive and arousing. Now let the wife lie on her back and the husband do the same, taking time to explore what feels best in the vagina as well as the labia and clitoris. Pull back the clitoral hood and notice the clitoris—massage to greater arousal and feel the clitoris become erect. Become a student of your mate's body.

# 3

# LOVEMAKING CYCLES

*R*eveling in a sexy atmosphere, the mounting excitement of the penis growing erect and the vagina lubricating in anticipation of intercourse, becoming playfully vulnerable and surrendering to orgasms stir up in each of us the passion and mystery of sexuality. God has designed a marvelously complex and intimate process to be set in motion when a couple make love.

A *process* can be defined as "a continuous series of changes over time." This chapter will develop two models of lovemaking cycles or processes with their evolving changes. The first, with Masters and Johnson, looks at the physical and bodily changes; while the second model, with Christopher McCluskey and his Lovemaking Cycle, considers the increasing emotional and relational intimacy during lovemaking.

Sex researchers Masters and Johnson developed from their research four separate phases of physical buildup and changes during sex: excitement, plateau, orgasm, and resolution. Understanding these phases can help couples enhance their arousal as they maximize each stage of the physical process.

## The Four-Phase Physical Process

### 1. The Excitement Phase

The husband's sexual excitement is a blend of physical friction in the erogenous zones and the mental arousal through sensual stimulation. Male arousal can be observed by the penis becoming erect. Remember that erections and vaginal lubrication can be reflexive and are not always indications of complete arousal. Erections are almost taken for granted until there are difficulties, but all men will struggle with getting or maintaining an erection at some point. Fatigue, alcohol, medications, and performance anxiety are common causes. The key is not to panic because that just compounds the problem. Create plenty of erotic stimulation and realize it is temporary.

Often during the excitement and plateau phases, the erection becomes partial/softer or completely subsides because the husband focuses on pleasuring his mate and has less direct penile stimulation. He also may get distracted and less focused and lose the erection. That is normal. As he enjoys the loveplay and erotic stimulation, the erection will return.

Female arousal in the excitement phase is demonstrated by vaginal lubrication, which is like beads of saliva that sweat through the outer walls of the vagina. This occurs within the first minute or two of arousal but can vary, especially with aging or distraction and an inability to focus on pleasure. The vaginal secretions have an odor much like saliva. Some foods (e.g., asparagus) will affect the odor of the secretions. The mind is a wonderful tool as it can pair the odors of making love (semen, vaginal secretions, perspiration) with sexual excitement and pleasure as they become exciting stimuli.

The nipples of the female become erect in the central papilla area during sexual excitement. The nipples, male and female, are a fun part of sexual loveplay. Within the vagina, the outer third becomes more engorged with blood (tumescent) during the excitement phase and is called the orgasmic platform. It is the most sensitive vaginal tissue, and stimulating the orgasmic platform feels great for both partners.

During arousal, the outer lips flatten and the inner lips of the vulva enlarge, creating a chute for the penis to travel down to the vagina. The clitoris enlarges to two or three times its relaxed size. This occurs under the skin at the clitoral hood and is not readily observable. It can be felt by rolling a finger over this area right above the clitoral hood, feeling much like a firm cord under the skin. Women vary immensely as to how they enjoy the clitoral stimulation, and this can change over the various phases. Keep talking. The wife may need to demonstrate how she prefers the clitoris to be stimulated.

## 2. The Plateau Phase

This phase should be the longest and perhaps the most enjoyable one of the sexual cycle. The initial arousal is there, and the loveplay can build on this tension as it progresses from general stimulation to specific locations. The penis becomes fuller and the head a deeper color as it is further engorged. The orgasmic platform in the outer third of the vagina also becomes larger, giving firmer friction on the penis during intercourse. The inner two-thirds of the vagina expands, creating a receptacle for the semen, and the uterus elevates, giving greater comfort with thrusting because the cervix is pulled away.

In the male, preparation for ejaculation is taking place as the prostate and seminal vesicles contract. Some seepage from the penis occurs; it does contain sperm, so be cautious to have birth control in place. In an ejaculation there are 250 to 500 million sperm, and it takes only one to create a baby. The seminal fluid is building in the urethra and area near the prostate, preparing for orgasm.

Both males and females experience increased heart rates; the blood pressure rises, and the breathing intensifies. With some, there is a sex flush on the upper torso, neck, and face. Muscles involuntarily contract, and sexual excitement continues to build gradually during this plateau phase. The loveplay will increase in intensity with active intercourse and more vigorous direct stimulation of the erogenous zones.

Research has found that a man, if actively thrusting, will often climax in less than two minutes while a woman will take longer to reach an orgasm. The wise couple intersperse intercourse and vary rhythms of thrusting throughout the plateau phase as the husband starts and stops and keeps his arousal on a plateau without peaking too soon. Both husband and wife can learn to approach an orgasm and then back off as they maintain the plateau phase for extended periods of pleasurable and sensuous lovemaking.

## 3. The Orgasm Phase

This phase focuses on producing an orgasm in one or both partners. The plateau phase has increased excitement, and now both partners are ready to climb that last peak with focused stimulation.

In allowing the reflexive action of an orgasm to occur, you must focus on your body and the tension that is building. Allow your mind to give in to the increasing arousal and revel in the approaching climax. At orgasm, you become self-focused and trust your partner with grimaces and squeals and muscle contractions. You are oblivious to how you look as your mind is selfishly centered on your growing excitement.

Physically, both the male and female experience muscle contractions, eight-tenths of a second in duration, as the central part of the orgasmic response. For the female, the contractions center in the vaginal area in the orgasmic platform with the PC (pubococcygeal) muscle and the rectal sphincter (circular muscle at the opening of the rectum). The uterus also contracts, much as in labor pains. The female experiences a series of spasms, four to twelve in duration depending on the intensity of the orgasm. The male experiences spasms during his ejaculation, which also vary in intensity depending on level of arousal and abandonment to the experience. His contractions occur around the prostate gland and along the seminal duct system and penis as the semen is propelled outward through the urethra.

With orgasm also come involuntary contractions of the muscles of the arms, legs, pelvis, and back. Breathing, blood pressure, and heart rate will increase. Sometimes deliberately stimulating these physiological aspects of an orgasm with tensing muscles and breathing heavily can trigger the climax.

There are interesting distinctions between male and female

orgasmic capabilities. Males have a refractory period, or recuperative time, between orgasms. At age nineteen, this rest period may be a few minutes; with aging, it increases to a few hours or days. The second orgasm following close to the first may take more stimulation and may be less intense.

Females, on the other hand, do not have a refractory period. They are capable of having repeated orgasms, and rather than diminish—succeeding orgasms may be more intense. Women may experience separate orgasms minutes apart, or during an intense lovemaking session with increasing arousal, they may experience them in rapid succession. This rapid succession may also be explained as a more intense orgasm, which can have ten to twelve spasms. Some women also experience a gushing of secretions and a greater wetness.

In the orgasm phase, a common concern is whether the wife should be able to climax during lovemaking by penile thrusting alone. Almost two-thirds of women can't achieve an orgasm without direct stimulation of the clitoris. Most wives will need manual or oral stimulation of the clitoris to create arousal up to the point of climaxing. Climaxing through intercourse could be likened to the husband having an orgasm by stroking his testicles but not his penis.

Remember that an orgasm is a reflexive response; it is not an intentional act of the will. You cannot consciously will yourself to have an orgasm. Orgasms are a product of sufficient buildup of physical, mental, and emotional stimulation as the mind focuses on that increasing sexual tension. For most women, the stimulation needs to be in the clitoral area where there is a concentration of nerve endings.

This is where the husband has to allow the wife to coach him as to what touches stimulate her best and what rhythm she desires. He controls his orgasm and rhythm by being the one thrusting his penis in her vagina—fast, slow, intensely, gently—however he desires. She is dependent on his hand, mouth, or penis to create the friction and buildup with the right touch, tempo, and building intensity.

Some women enjoy their orgasms with the penis in the vagina and experience greater intensity, while some prefer not to have the penis in the vagina as they focus on their own sensations. Some couples like orgasms close together, and others prefer allowing a woman to climax several times before the man. Create the patterns and rhythms that fit you as an individual and as a couple.

## 4. THE RESOLUTION PHASE

After an orgasm, both men and women experience a release of tension as the body returns to its original state before sexual arousal. This is physically the final enjoyment of an orgasm as the muscles relax, blood vessels and tissue release the engorged blood, and the congestion abruptly eases. Sometimes with men and women, the genitals become very sensitive after an orgasm.

There is a feeling of tension release with an orgasm as the blood congestion leaves the genital, pelvic area with a pleasant, perhaps tingling, sensation. In the woman, unlike the man, there is the potential to return quite quickly to an aroused state and experience multiple orgasms. The wife may learn to experience several orgasms as she then returns to the plateau phase with her husband. It can be fulfilling for both of them.

Spend time allowing the body to enjoy each of the four phases as you cycle through excitement, plateau, orgasm, and resolution. In becoming an expert lover, the right-hand graph is more pleasurable, especially for the wife, than the left-hand graph and more characteristic of a fun lovemaking session.

Figure 2.5
The four phases of arousal and satisfaction: frustrated (left) and fulfilled

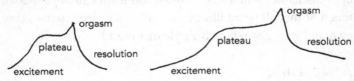

## THE LOVEMAKING CYCLE

While Masters and Johnson focus on four phases of physical arousal, Christian sex therapist Christopher McCluskey has created a more relational and emotional Lovemaking Cycle. He insists that there is a great deal of difference between having sex and making love. True lovemaking (the Cycle) creates a growing intimacy and an increasing sexual passion based on two hearts who are becoming spiritually and emotionally one.

In McCluskey's model, each part of the cycle feeds into the next, creating an ever-deepening experience of vulnerability and intimacy with your mate and lover. He emphasizes that if one part is neglected, lovemaking will "clunk" every time it hits that weak spot and throw off the whole cycle—much like a wheel that is flat in one area and no longer round. Lovemaking will in time break down because each of the four parts represents a deep emotional and relational need that is critical for maintaining passionate lovemaking.

This model identifies many important factors that can facilitate progressively deeper levels of intimacy in lovemaking. Each will be briefly examined and explained with an emphasis on the four key areas that are truly interactive and must flow from the heart: atmosphere, arousal, apex, and afterglow. (A brief disclaimer is in order. Though this is McCluskey's model, much of the following illustrative and descriptive matter is my own and may not reflect his style or values.)

## ATMOSPHERE

Mood-setting is not simply lighting a candle or creating a

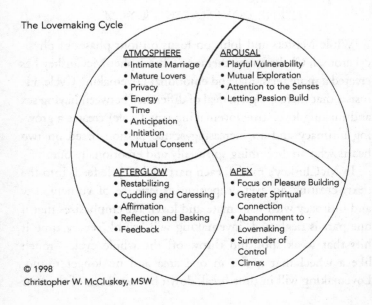

The Lovemaking Cycle

ATMOSPHERE
- Intimate Marriage
- Mature Lovers
- Privacy
- Energy
- Time
- Anticipation
- Initiation
- Mutual Consent

AROUSAL
- Playful Vulnerability
- Mutual Exploration
- Attention to the Senses
- Letting Passion Build

AFTERGLOW
- Restabilizing
- Cuddling and Caressing
- Affirmation
- Reflection and Basking
- Feedback

APEX
- Focus on Pleasure Building
- Greater Spiritual Connection
- Abandonment to Lovemaking
- Surrender of Control
- Climax

© 1998
Christopher W. McCluskey, MSW

little ambience. *The concept of atmosphere is much deeper.* It is lovingly building an intimate relationship with your covenant companion so that energy is reserved and time is devoted for sexuality. Time, energy, and anticipation are powerful aphrodisiacs. Desire is never just hormonal, especially for the wife. Sex begins with loving attention in the kitchen and flows into passion in the bedroom. Lovers anticipate each other, and sexual passion permeates the relationship regardless of place or circumstances.

*Intimate marriage and mature lovers.* This goes back to the formula for fulfilling and passionate sexual encounters. The foundation of fantastic lovemaking is an intimate, grown-up companionship that includes effective communication.

*Privacy.* God designed sexual intimacy to be a very special and private interaction between husband and wife. Though making love should not be confined to the bedroom, it will be the primary love nest because of the need for privacy as well as for comfort. Mood lighting or candles, sensuous linens, and the ability to control the temperature are sexual enhancements that can give the bedroom very private, sensual, and erotic qualities. You can also create an intimate privacy in other parts of your home and in that hotel room on your honeymoon. It is just the two of you alone.

*Energy.* Even if you are newlyweds, you will have to reserve some energy for sex. Can you remember how exhausted you were on your honeymoon night? Think of what rest and a boost of energy would have done. Putting some extra current into your love life will have a marvelous effect.

*Time.* If five minutes is great, then forty-five will be even more intimate. Time may be the most precious gift you bring to your sex life. It is the bottom line in creating the sexy, connected atmosphere as you get beyond quickies to luxuriating. Five-second hugs, lingering-deep kisses, and two-hour picnics in bed will do wonders.

*Anticipation.* Great lovers are childlike in their ability to anticipate pleasure with glee. Husbands and especially wives can enjoy their God-given imagination and think about lovemaking more—like a kid who has looked forward to the ice cream store all day. Anticipation also has a deeper quality of mentally preparing your bodies and spirits to being truly naked and vulnerable.

*Initiation.* Lovemaking has to start somewhere, and a part of ambience is both husband and wife initiating sexual activity. Initiation does not have to lead to intercourse but can be that passionate kiss when arriving home from work. Grow into verbal as well as nonverbal forms of initiating. Verbal can be even more intimate.

*Mutual consent.* If you want to maintain a great mood for sex, be *assertive* and *empathetic* in your intimate communication. Lovemaking is about giving and not demanding. You aren't trying to service each other. The husband or the wife may not be in the mood and that's okay, but what great fireworks happen when you do mutually engage!

## AROUSAL
Sexual maturity helps us grow beyond the arousal of sexual rushes and buzzes. Deep, erotic arousal grows from a three-dimensional (body, soul, spirit) connection and bonding.

When you and your mate learn to be aroused in a truly *intimate* way, you will be amazed at the feelings that occur. The physical and emotional interaction and fusion (God-given *eros*) create an unbeatable intimacy high.

*Playful vulnerability.* Fun and open lovemaking takes place in the child ego state. Each of us has that curious, silly, innocent, playful part of us that loves to romp. "Naked and unashamed" is a very vulnerable yet powerful place to be.

Couples sometimes worry that certain props (like lingerie or body oils) create artificial or sinfully seductive arousal and will detract from their natural lovemaking. I strongly believe that God gave imaginations to create and enjoy various means of enticing and playing with our mates. Props can enhance experiences and sensations. Flickering candlelight with soothing music in the background creates totally different feelings from those created by mirrors employed in an afternoon delight with some jazz on the stereo. Pillows as props are great to lean against as you have intimate conversations or to use in positions of pleasuring and intercourse. They help make the bed the playground it should be. A great rule of thumb about props is that they (1) remain playfully in perspective, (2) not detract from your vulnerability and respect, (3) enhance true three-dimensional (body, soul, and spirit) passion.

*Mutual exploration.* Many mates have never taken the time to examine each other's genitals and familiarize themselves with the hot spots. Take the time to truly be present with each other in curious, teasing, and exploratory ways. The Song of Solomon delightfully encourages lovers to "browse among the lilies."

*Attention to the senses.* Every couple can wisely make two

lists. The first list is of each of the five senses and how each sense can cue you in to sexual arousal—how you want that sense to be utilized. The second list is what turns you off with each sense and detracts from lovemaking. A sample list:

*Sight.* Turn-ons: Show up naked. A couple holding hands. Strategically placed mirrors. Seductive dances. Bright satin sheets. Emerald boxers. Soft peach teddies. Turn-offs: Bright lights. A beer gut. The same nightgown. Dirty sheets.

*Smell.* Turn-ons: Perfumes, candles, incense, scented lotions. Semen. Bubble bath. Turn-offs: Semen. Body odor. Dirty sheets. Dragon breath.

*Taste.* Turn-ons: Chocolate and strawberries. Minty kisses. A favorite wine. Turn-offs: Certain lubricants. Garlic kisses.

*Hearing.* Turn-ons: Favorite songs. Sexy talking. Uninhibited groans and squeals. Turn-offs: Squeals in ear. Silence. Television. Slang.

*Touch.* Turn-ons: Soaping each other up. Ice cubes over sensitive areas. A fur rug. Satin gloves (fabrics are sensual). Lotions. Sweaty bodies rubbing. Turn-offs: Unshaven beards. Rough hands. Sweaty bodies. Tickling.

*Letting passion build.* Arousal carries with it the idea of a crescendo and increasing excitement. In a mature way, you are responsible for your own passionate feelings. A healthy self-focus is important in letting passions build. Get into your private feelings and share them with your mate. What a powerful turn-on as you build toward the apex.

## APEX

It takes a mature person to understand that the emotional center of the apex is not orgasm, but a surrender to feelings and each other. The term "apex" is purposefully used to de-emphasize chasing orgasms and to emphasize the deeper idea of abandonment and achieving a deeper oneness. Most often there will be that exciting climax, but there will be some times when an orgasm will not occur and yet an apex is achieved. Mature, older couples have often grown into this level of apex and enjoy its beauty.

*Focus on pleasure building.* Remember that women vary more in what they find pleasurable, and the center of sensory nerves for them is the clitoris and not the vagina. Stay in the moment with a growing focus on accenting what each partner is experiencing.

*Greater spiritual connection.* Look deeply into each other's eyes and get lost in each other and the sharing of passion. Lovemaking can make you more totally "naked" than any other mutual experience. Your emotions and your bodies are making heavenly music that is much more profound than the friction.

*Abandonment to lovemaking.* Only with commitment and trust do you feel safe enough to abandon yourself to another person. Your covenant companionship provides that context. You no longer need to be self-conscious but can be passionate without any inhibitions. You are unconditionally loved and accepted.

*Surrender of control.* This is the heart of the apex and indeed of becoming orgasmic. Orgasms are such beautiful metaphors of uninhibited worship and giving up control to Christ. You are allowing your bodies and souls to soar with surrender.

*Climax.* You lose time and your body and feelings overwhelm the rational. What a precious gift to share with that lifetime lover—again and again with ever-increasing meaning and passion.

## AFTERGLOW

The lovemaking wheel will begin clunking if lovers neglect this important stage. It may last three to five minutes or an hour, but this time is critical for maintaining sexual passion. The afterglow—regrouping, complimenting, evaluating, and an anticipation of the next occurrence of lovemaking—fuels the fire and greases the wheel.

*Restabilizing.* After the apex you need to catch your breath and come down physically and emotionally. This is the afterglow that is warmly intimate but less intense. A time of re-creating and affirming the recently shared intimate moment is needed.

*Cuddling and caressing.* Wives are especially vulnerable after literally opening themselves up to their husbands. Rather than jumping up to clean up, hold each other and bask in the afterglow of intense connecting and shared surrender. Affirm the closeness.

*Affirmation.* Husbands so want to please their wives and be great lovers. A "Wow, I can't believe what you just did" goes really far at this point. The wife wants to feel sexy and valued; compliments are important to her too. Not "Great butt," but "It's awesome how your body makes me irrational." Mates soak up praise and compliments.

*Reflection and basking.* Wives often comment how their husbands will engage in connecting conversation after love-making more than any other time. You have become vulnerably close. Reflect and bask in the relationship as well as in the events of the past moments.

*Feedback.* Feedback can start the wheel rolling for the next lovemaking session. "Let's do that again" or "Could we make love Thursday morning?" This is indeed an ongoing party, and you are enriching and preparing for the next festivity.

Isn't lovemaking exciting?! You will be learning new pleasures fifty years from now. Keep tuning in to all four aspects—atmosphere, arousal, apex, and afterglow—so the wheel of your love life doesn't clunk and you can experience the ever-increasing passion God designed.

(Note: Christopher McCluskey and his wife, Rachel, have written a forthcoming book on the Lovemaking Cycle with Baker/Revell Publishers. He also has an excellent videotape, *Coaching Couples into Passionate Intimacy,* which explains the model and can be ordered through his Web site at www.christian-living.com.)

TIME OUT . . .

1. Discuss your turn-ons and turn-offs in these areas: sight, smell, taste, hearing, touch.

2. What gets in the way of really surrendering to your climaxes? Discuss this together. While making love and the apex approaches, pretend you are on a roller-coaster ride and trust your mate as you truly surrender to this ride and its out-of-control feelings.

## 4

# EROTIC PLEASURING

*B*ecoming lovers is fun work. This chapter focuses on the sensual pleasuring of your mate's body and genitals as a bonding part of making love. Nondemanding genital pleasuring does not mean you must exclude orgasms. It simply means that erotic, passionate sexual touching can be hampered if it is always goal-oriented toward rushing into intercourse or producing a climax. Wives, if you have not experienced an orgasm, that is a needed goal (cf. Chapter 10), and pleasuring can be a fun part of achieving that objective.

*Pleasure* is an interesting word. Somehow it almost does not seem to fit within Christian values. It feels self-centered and sinful. The truth of the matter is that God gave us our sensuality to enjoy. The sin is not in experiencing pleasure but in calling pleasure sinful and not allowing ourselves to enjoy God's many gifts, including erotic sensuality. I've known Christians to worry about the word *erotic*. The Greek word *eros* portrays the idea of passion, chemistry and fusion, a magnetic field with a strong attraction. One-flesh lovers are erotic in the best and strongest sense of the word.

Enjoying physical pleasuring that is slow and bonding without pressure and demands is critical to a truly intimate, nurturing, and exciting sex life. You need to be able to make love for half an hour to a couple of hours at a time. Pleasuring can be a focused, sensual massage as you luxuriate and focus in on your sensuality and sexuality. It requires that you notice and give yourself permission to enjoy your sexual feelings. Telling your mate what you like and not being afraid to ask for more is an important part of this process. Sensuous, playful mates find it exciting to include erogenous loveplay in their repertoire of bonding activities.

## POSITIONS FOR EROTIC PLEASURING

Here are two relaxing and comfortable positions that lend themselves to nondemanding erotic pleasuring of various kinds. In each position, you may wish to lie on pillows or use the back of the bed to prop up and get comfortable.

The greatest source of male sexual arousal is the head of the penis, while female arousal is centered in the clitoris. During intercourse the penis is being constantly stimulated—but the clitoris isn't. With these nondemanding positions of pleasuring, the Level Two erogenous zones and the genitals are easily accessible. The hands are free to caress and massage both genital and nongenital areas as your souls and bodies communicate. Again, be sure sensitive tissue is lubricated, which can increase the sensuality.

### 1. SITTING OR LYING WITH LEGS OVERLAPPED

The pleasuring position of sitting with legs overlapped allows better availability to the most sensitive parts of the male and female anatomies. You can experiment with which legs are better on top in the overlapping process and what level of being prone helps. The pleasuree may wish to lie flat with knees bent and focus on personal pleasure, or both may wish to face each other sitting. This position lends itself to communicating and exchanging nonverbal signs of pleasure. Here are possible uses of this position for the wife and husband as she or he is the genital pleasurer.

*Wife as pleasurer.* Sit with legs overlapping (whichever is most comfortable) and your husband sitting or lying flat. His buttocks and genitals are almost in your lap. Start with caressing his face, chest, stomach, and thighs—connect with him physically. As you continue to do this with one hand, take your other hand and play with his testicles and penis. Now direct your full attention to the penis. Have him close his eyes and revel in the sensations as you run your fingers up and down and stroke the shaft and head. Build the excitement as you use the stimulation that can create a climax. As he approaches an

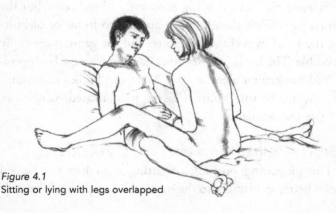

Figure 4.1
Sitting or lying with legs overlapped

orgasm, stop your active stroking of the penis and let his arousal slow down.

Now direct your attention to yourself as you use his penis as a wand to stimulate your genital area. You may need a pillow under your buttocks or for one of you to lie more prone as you match up genital areas. He may lose some of his arousal, but that is good as you prolong this pleasuring session. He will enjoy your continued penile touching as well as learning what strokes and rhythms are arousing to you. This is a vulnerable mutual sharing of sexual feelings. Go slow at first, and stimulate your whole vulval area as you keep coming back to the clitoris. Bring yourself to a climax first if you so desire, then focus back on his sensations and build him to an orgasm.

*Husband as the pleasurer.* With your wife almost sitting in your lap, start with a hug, and caress her back and face, sucking her fingers and lightly kissing her arms, running your fingers teasingly over her breasts and stomach as you approach and back off from the nipples. You are arousing and connecting with your lover before approaching direct genital stimulation. As she becomes aroused and desires more genital excitement, have her lie back with her legs continuing to overlap yours. Arouse your penis to a full erection, and use it to slowly stimulate the whole vulval area as you spread her lips apart and lightly caress. Lovers find the penis is a marvelous tool for stimulating the clitoral area.

As she becomes more aroused, use your penis to increase the stimulation of the clitoris. Let her guide you in what area feels best and what motions are more arousing. As you use your wrist and arm to create vibrating sensations, you can also stroke the shaft of the penis as a part of these motions, continuing to also increase your sexual buildup. Be creative as you vibrate faster, then slow down some; apply lighter pressure and more direct pressure; turn your penis down to the vagina and back up to the clitoris. Entice and tease as you take plenty of time to enjoy each other and slowly build to a climax. After she has had an orgasm, you can bring yourself to one, also.

## 2. SITTING WITH BACK TO CHEST

This position has the pleasuree sitting comfortably between the legs of the pleasurer, leaning back against his or her chest to be cuddled and pleasured. The hands of the pleasurer have access to the face, chest, abdomen, and genitals of the partner. The pleasurer can be propped up against the back of the bed for comfort. An important part of nondemanding erotic pleasuring is feeling close and connected as you sensuously enjoy your mate's body, as well as give him or her pleasure. This position allows special closeness as you cuddle up close to your

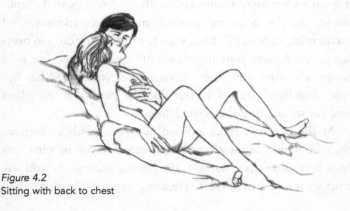

Figure 4.2
Sitting with back to chest

partner and enjoy the delight of the hands. Another important aspect of mutual pleasuring is feeling supported and comfortable physically. This position helps prevent aching backs and sore knees.

## COACHING THE EROTIC PLEASURE

Teaching your mate what feels sensual and arousing to you is critical. Utilize several of the pleasuring positions as you alternate blocks of pleasuring time. This will challenge you as a couple in many growth-producing ways. It will require you to tune in to your own pleasure as you instruct your mate about what you desire and find stimulating. It will perfect your coaching techniques: verbally, in talking about what you desire; and nonverbally, in guiding hand and illustrating motions. You may need to put your hand over your mate's hand and actually demonstrate the strokes, pressure, and rhythms that you enjoy. You will become more comfortable in asking for what you want and demonstrating your desires. These are vital skills for a great sex life over the next fifty years.

## THE PLEASURE OF ORAL STIMULATION

In the same way that kissing and intimately sharing mouths bring erotic arousal and intimate bonding, oral stimulation of the genitals can build trust and be exciting for mates. A quick bath and good hygiene are crucial for this genital pleasuring. If seepage bothers you, keep a warm washcloth handy and gently wipe as needed. Don't worry about his climaxing in your mouth—you as wife are assertive and can verbalize what you do and don't want. Actively share your needs and sensibilities.

Remember that Scripture is silent on the topic of oral sex. You as mates will have to sort and pray through certain behaviors as you choose what to include in your repertoire of love-making. Never make your mate feel guilty or inhibited because he or she does not feel comfortable with a given behavior. The object is to be playful, lovingly connected, and creatively varied. This can be accomplished without oral sex.

Trusting your genitals to your mate's mouth is warmly intimate. The genitals are called the "privates" for a reason. Husbands are very protective of the penis and testicles. To allow the partner complete access is an important commitment as they feel very vulnerable and in turn, arousingly close. Wives have sometimes bought into the notion that somehow they are dirty down there, or they have left their genitals as an unknown area. To have the husband intimately scrutinizing and enjoying this part of the body takes special trust and openness.

Here are a few suggestions for wife and husband to enhance this variety of genital pleasuring:

Wife, use your lips as buffers for your teeth in order to prevent damage to sensitive tissue. Use tongue and mouth to tease as you manually stoke the shaft of the penis and create firmer stimulation. Allow your mouth to create a vacuum effect—the stronger the sucking action, the more pleasurable the feelings produced. The head of the penis is the most sensitive part—don't worry about trying to take more of the penis into your mouth.

Husband, tease with your tongue as you flick it lightly over the vulval area. Kiss and gently suck the entire area. If your tongue gets tired, hold it firm and create rubbing sensations by moving your entire head side to side. You can also create sucking motions with your mouth over the clitoris to produce a climax. Keep teeth covered and employ variety until she actively approaches an orgasm.

Oral sex can be interspersed with other types of genital pleasuring in a nondemanding, emotionally connecting manner. It can be more exciting at times if combined with simultaneous manual stimulation. While enjoying oral sex, keep your hands active, too, as penis and testicles are stroked, fingers are inserted in vagina, back is caressed, buttocks are massaged, and skin is teased. Inhibition vanishes and control is relaxed as partners revel in each other's sensuality and sexuality.

Genital pleasuring may not come easily to you or feel comfortable. You may need practice in tuning in to the pleasurable sensations of your body and allowing excitement to build. Let go of your embarrassment, need for control, or fears and relax in the excitement of mutual pleasuring. You are creating a special intimacy.

In this discussion on genital pleasuring, some important issues need to be discussed by every couple. What do we do with masturbation? I am not talking about stimulating yourself during the course of mutual lovemaking. In some positions of intercourse the wife can more easily reach her clitoris. I'm referring to masturbation as an activity done alone to produce a climax and release. The Bible is neutral on masturbation, but 1 Corinthians 6:12 exhorts, "All things are lawful for me, but all things are not helpful." If you are masturbating, it is saying something about your intimacy or lack of it. One husband whose job included 60 percent travel struggled with masturbating. He resolved to quit masturbating on the road, and they made love within a day of his leaving and coming back. He related how it helped him keep his thought life on track and carry through on God's desire for sex to be intimate.

Can the person with the higher need for sexual activity have his or her needs met without the total participation of the partner? One wife told her husband that some nights she could honor that he needed sex more than she did and nurture him through to an orgasm. He refused because this seemed like pity or duty sex and that did not seem very fun or fair. She told him that she was assertive enough to say "no" if it was just an obligation. They ended up with some quickies with intercourse and other times manually achieving release with his caressing her breasts and both being naked and close.

Keep balance in your lovemaking, and don't just focus on intercourse and orgasm. This may seem odd advice when the next chapter is completely focused on intercourse, but marital partners need to play together in a variety of ways.

# 5

# CREATIVE INTERCOURSE

$\mathcal{U}$nleashing a childlike curiosity, becoming delightfully uninhibited, trying new things, and being playmates are all part of this vital component of exciting intercourse. Your imaginations and relationship can take these uninspired techniques and bring them alive. Some practice and experimenting can create great variety and immense romantic pleasure.

PLAYFUL, CREATIVE SENSUALITY + KNOWLEDGE +
PRACTICE = CREATIVE INTERCOURSE

You as a lover provide the fusion, sensuality, and excitement to intercourse. You as a couple can choose when and where you want to enjoy these positions, whether on a soft mattress, under the stars, or in the shower. You control the candlelight, music, lotions, lubrication, and ambience.

## PLAYFUL, CREATIVE SENSUALITY

Enjoy the total array of your senses and lovingly enhance touch as you employ the suggestions and encouragement of earlier chapters. Go slow and build tension as you sensuously progress through the lovemaking process. You can enjoy intercourse in different ways during the arousal and plateau phases of the sexual cycle. Let intercourse and various positions be interspersed throughout the arousal activities as you warmly connect as well as build tension. Each position will offer a new variety of ways to stimulate, touch, and take pleasure from each other's bodies. Allow your hands and mouth to keep actively caressing and stroking throughout intercourse. Focus on yourself and your partner.

## KNOWLEDGE AND PRACTICE

Becoming a great technical lover in intercourse is more than just knowing physiology and the various positions. The actual entry of the penis into the vagina can be new and exciting every time. Intercourse and the bonding one-flesh experience of lovers joining bodies should be an emotional and mental rush. Slow your mind and focus on the actual physical feelings of entry; don't take it routinely. As one partner separates the outer vulval lips and guides the penis in, each can delight again in the other's body. Over the many years together, this scintillating connection you enjoy can have a delightful electricity every time you experience it anew.

Make sure the lubrication (artificial or the seepage at the tip of the penis) has been gently spread over the head of the penis and the vaginal lubrication has wet the mouth of the vagina. (Dry skin chafes and hurts; be sure the vagina is lubricated.) The husband should take care not to simply shove in and start vigorously thrusting. Part the outer lips, and position the penis at the mouth of the vagina or allow the penis to sensually slide down the inner labial channel to the vagina. Slowly and gently push the penis in, reveling in the sensations. Slowly thrust partway in a time or two with tender gentleness as lubrication is spread, and revel in the feelings. Perhaps lightly shove the penis all the way in and start to thrust, while the husband wiggles his penis by using his PC muscle and while the wife tightens her PC muscle; feel warm and close in this one-flesh embrace. Allow the vagina to lovingly contain its partner.

Practice different rhythms of coital thrusting with pelvic muscles as both partners push to meet each other or one controls a given movement. The outer third of the vagina is particularly sensitive—the husband can practice quick, shallow thrusting at the mouth of the vagina, flicking the penis in and out. The stimulation and arousal caused by the angle and depth of the penis penetrating the vagina will vary from woman to woman. Talk and experiment. Varying the position will create different angles or allow deeper penetration. Enjoy what is exciting to you.

With intercourse, as with all sexual activity, enjoyment and passion will be enhanced by your imaginations and stored erotic stimuli. Certain positions can excite the visual sense of the husband, and others the romantic, connecting needs of the wife. Invent a fun repertoire together. Men, remember that this has nothing to do with the size of your penis. As the country saying goes, "It is not the depth of the well, or the *length of the rope*—it's how you dangle the bucket." Wives, remember that most women do not experience orgasms just with intercourse but need more direct clitoral stimulation. Celebrate the bonding, nurturing, and excitement of intercourse. It is indeed a fun playground activity for the loving, creative couple. At times, forgo any movement and just lie in each other's arms, basking in the warmth of one-flesh togetherness.

## EIGHT TYPES OF INTERCOURSE POSITIONS

You know the old saying that "practice makes perfect." Any new position will be awkward at first and perhaps not as fun, warmly connecting, or erotically arousing as ones you are used to. Practice is important so that you as a couple can quickly begin to enjoy different positions in an adept and relaxed manner. They say that if you use new vocabulary words three times in your conversation, they are yours for life. Do this with the following positions of intercourse too.

Relax and play at acquiring this knowledge. Be creative as you make up some of your own variations to try. Also, practice shifting into a new position from an existing position without removing the penis. Men and women have different physical and psychological makeups and will have differing preferences about what is exciting to them. Be sensitive to each other as you take this knowledge and give it playful, creative sensuality.

### 1. WIFE-ON-TOP

The wife-on-top positions are favorites for several reasons. For the husband who has a bad back or knees, this position takes the pressure off and allows his wife to be the active participant. It is also the needed position for a couple with disabilities who want to press into the vagina the flaccid penis of the husband. The positions are visually very arousing to the male, and the female is more in control of her own stimulation. Many women find being on top positions the vagina and clitoris to achieve orgasm more readily during intercourse. The husband's hands are also nicely placed to stimulate the clitoris as needed.

*Kneeling.* The wife kneels while she straddles her husband. She can use a number of angles: a backward tilt as she supports herself with arms straight and hands on his legs or the bed, a 90-degree upright stance with bouncing motions, or a 45-degree forward tilt with weight on arms or forearms propped on pillows. This position allows the woman to control the depth of penile penetration and orchestrate the movement of the penis in the vagina with the clitoris against the pelvic bone. It may be easier for her to guide the penis into the vagina. It is also pleasurable to simply lay the penis on his stomach and, with proper lubrication, rub the clitoral area back and forth with a rocking motion across the erect penis without vaginal penetration.

The husband can also thrust with pelvic motions. This

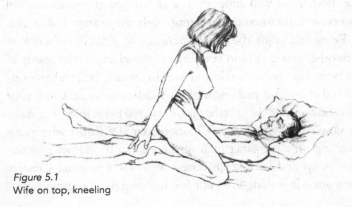

Figure 5.1
Wife on top, kneeling

position is fun for the husband because his wife's breasts are near his face and mouth, and the pubic area is very visible. The wife can enjoy the easy access her husband has to massage the clitoris with his thumb. For variation and different sensations, the wife can kneel facing away from the husband.

*Prone.* The wife lies comfortably on top with her legs straddling his body or between his legs, finding leverage with her feet and knees. She may also wish to prop her shins and feet insteps on top of her husband's lower legs and hold her feet against his feet to gain leverage for giving thrusting motions. In this prone position, as well as others, it is easier to insert the penis in a corollary position (wife kneeling) and then ease into the position desired. The woman-on-top position allows the wife to take the lead in a fun, selfish way, using her husband's body for her pleasure.

## 2. SIDE-BY-SIDE

Couples enjoy side-by-side positions because bodies are comfortably close and facing each other for cuddling and kissing. Bodies are well supported, and both partners can control and contribute to coital thrusting while they caress and stroke.

Relax and enjoy the total experience of intercourse. Look at each other and delight in your mate's arousal and in the beauty of the body. Gently caress skin and revel in texture. Talk and give verbal and nonverbal exchanges of love and excitement. Close your eyes and focus on the specific pleasure of the penis in the vagina— go slow with light, feathery motions, rapidly thrust with penis touching only the outer inch of the vagina, try deeper penetration—stop and lie in each other's arms for a minute. Creative intercourse is making love, not just building to an orgasm.

Figure 5.2
Side-by-side, wife straddling
husband's leg

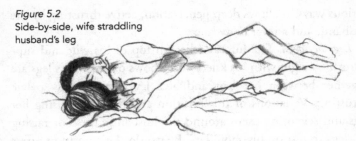

*Wife straddling husband's leg.* The husband lies comfortably on his side, with his bottom leg extended straight, his other leg bent at the knee, and his foot on the bed. The wife lies on her side and straddles the top bent leg, with her lower leg between his legs and her top leg thrown over his torso. This positions the penis at the vagina (with proper shifting) for easy access with either partner guiding it in. Again, pillows under heads or sides increase comfort.

*Couple embracing chest to chest.* The wife lies on her side with the husband facing her in a mutual embrace. This may be most easily achieved by rolling over onto the sides from the wife-on-top or husband-on-top positions. The husband's top arm and hand are free to caress his wife's buttocks and back. This can be a fun, bonding embrace as you adjust the underneath arms for greatest comfort and both supply movement.

## 3. HUSBAND-ON-TOP

This has often been called the missionary position because, according to legend, the Hawaiians did not employ this position as the missionaries did. This standard position is often thought of as uncreative or elementary. Actually, it is pleasurable in various ways. It allows deep penetration, active thrusting by the husband, and a total body hug.

*Legs between.* The husband lies on top of his wife and supports his weight with his knees and elbows or arms. His legs are together between her legs and give leverage for easy pelvic thrusting. Variations of this position are the wife's raising her legs and scissoring them around the husband's torso or raising her legs to rest on his shoulders. Be gentle. This position offers perhaps the deepest penetration of any position.

*Legs straddling.* It is easier for the husband to start with legs together and the penis inserted in the vagina. Now, with the penis remaining inserted, he can gently shift one of his legs outside one of his wife's legs as he straddles that leg. For different sensations, he can shift his other leg from between to outside as he straddles with both legs outside his wife's legs. This allows his wife to clamp or scissor her legs together and produce greater friction on the penis in her vagina. The husband has an easy swinging motion of the pelvis and can raise up on his knees and elbows to relieve any excess pressure on his wife.

The husband-on-top position gives an ability to be body to body in a special one-flesh hug. Try just lying there in an intercourse embrace, remembering your commitment and love for each other as you rest warmly, savoring your togetherness.

## 4. CROSSWISE

Both crosswise positions are great for freeing hands to stimulate the clitoris and caress bodies. While the husband is thrusting, the wife can caress his testicles or scissor two of her fingers around his thrusting penis to increase stimulation. She can also stimulate herself or hold his hand as he stimulates her clitoral area. The husband can maneuver his body (collapsing the + into an X) while keeping the penis in the vagina so that he is able to nibble at her breasts and enjoy kissing, too, in these positions.

*Wife's legs over.* The husband lies on his side facing the wife, crosswise on the bed. His wife lies on her back and creates a cross of their bodies by resting her legs over his thighs with one leg toward his waist and the other leg toward his knees, allowing easy penetration by the penis. The husband creates the thrusting motion with pelvic movement.

*Scissors.* The husband lies crosswise on the bed with his head to the wife's right, and she lies on her back. This time the wife's right leg is propped over her husband's thighs, and her left leg is scissored between her husband's legs. If the husband is left-handed, he scissors her right leg, placing his head on her left side. This leaves manipulation and penetration of the penis to be controlled easily by the husband.

Scissors is an ideal position for using the penis as a wand to stimulate the vulva and clitoris. The husband can hold his

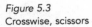
Figure 5.3
Crosswise, scissors

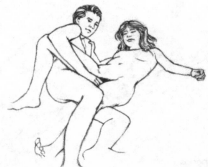

erect penis and, with the wife's instructions, learn the right rhythms and pressure and placement to help her achieve an orgasm. If the wrist grows tired, he can use more of the entire arm, like painting, to vibrate and massage the clitoris. This can be interspersed with vaginal thrusting to keep the whole area lubricated. As she approaches a climax, the husband may wish to switch to vaginal stimulation alone.

Either crosswise position works well during pregnancy. From the scissors position, the couple can maneuver into the next position without withdrawing the penis. The wife rolls on her side with her back toward the husband. The husband gently unscissors her leg, then slides his legs so they are behind hers in a spoon position as he thrusts against her buttocks.

## 5. REAR-ENTRY

The rear-entry positions, especially the lying-down spoons or both kneeling on the bed, are great during pregnancy. The wife should be comfortably supported with pillows as needed, and thrusting should be as gentle as desired.

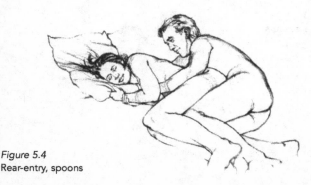

Figure 5.4
Rear-entry, spoons

*Spoons.* The husband faces his wife's back, like two spoons cradling. The penis can be inserted with the husband separating legs and outer vulval lips, while the wife guides the penis into the vagina. Male pelvic thrusting bumps softly against her buttocks as the penis stimulates the front of the vagina and the G spot.

The husband can enjoy caressing his wife's stomach and breasts and stimulating her clitoris with his free hand. The wife often likes this angle of the penis with slow or vigorous thrusting that is exciting but not too deep. Both are comfortable with less demand on muscles and joints.

*Kneeling in husband's lap.* The husband kneels with knees together and back upright. The wife kneels with her back to him, straddling his legs and propping herself in his lap—carefully inserting the penis as a mutual effort. He can place his hands on her hips to help control movement as she moves up and down, and he can create some pelvic thrusting. She may wish to bend forward and brace herself with her arms. This position leaves the husband's hands free to caress, while the wife can control depth and positioning of the penis with pelvic and leg movements.

*Both kneeling.* The husband kneels behind his wife, who is kneeling, bent at the waist with forearms and head resting comfortably on a pillow or the edge of the bed. The husband separates the outer lips from the rear and gently inserts his penis into the vagina. This position may seem awkward to the wife, but it is very visually stimulating to the husband. He has an exciting view of waist and hips and his penis penetrating the vulval area. It also allows easy thrusting motions from slow to vigorous and stimulation of the sensitive twelve o'clock part of the vagina.

Another variant of this position is for the wife to slide down into a prone position on the bed, with a pillow under her stomach propping up her buttocks and genital area. The husband lies down on her back with his legs between her legs and inserts his penis. He can get leverage for thrusting with his feet and knees as he hugs her from the back.

## 6. STANDING

The standing positions encourage creative intercourse without the need for a bed. They are fun for rooms of the house other than the bedroom.

*From the back.* This is similar to both kneeling, only both partners are standing. The wife bends at the waist and supports her weight with her hands on a bed, a table, or shower fixtures.

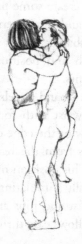

Figure 5.5
Standing, facing
with wife on one leg

The husband stands or crouches behind her and, separating the outer labia with one hand, inserts the penis. This can be a fun position for a quickie in the kitchen or a romp in the shower.

*Facing with wife on one leg.* The wife faces the husband and raises her left leg, which he cradles with his right hand, and they mutually insert the penis. If the husband is much taller than the wife, she may need to stand on a small stool or pillow. This position permits eye-to-eye contact and a chance to mutually hug and caress.

## 7. FACE-TO-FACE

These face-to-face positions will remind you of the wife-on-top and the rear-entry kneeling (only reversed) positions of intercourse. The fun comes in as you stay creatively sensual and are willing to experiment. As playfulness and curiosity take over, you can create many hybrids on your own.

*Husband sitting and wife kneeling.* The husband sits upright with his back propped against pillows, while his wife kneels astride his lap facing him with her legs around his thighs. This position allows for fun hugging and kissing and looking into each other's eyes. It provides close body contact but not much leverage for thrusting. Movement can be assisted by the husband's hands under his wife's buttocks and bouncing motions. The penis can be mutually inserted, and since this position allows for deep penetration, care must be taken for comfort. This is a good position if the husband has back problems because he can be comfortable with his back propped with pillows.

*Wife supine and husband kneeling.* The husband kneels and his wife, lying on her back, places her legs over his thighs with

Figure 5.6
Face-to-face, wife supine
and husband kneeling

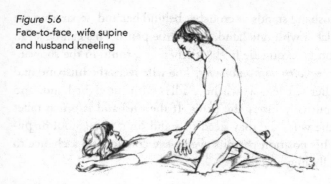

knees bent and feet flat on the bed. It may help to prop a pillow under her head and shoulders or position a pillow under her buttocks to position the penis better. This is a good position for using the penis to stimulate the clitoris. If the angle is too much to allow easy penetration, the husband may wish to bend forward and cradle his wife's legs with his hands under her buttocks or waist so access is more comfortable. This allows pelvic thrusting as well as adjustments and movement with his arms. Again, husband and wife are face-to-face so they can enjoy each other visually. (For variety, have the wife flip over on her stomach with the insteps of her feet on the husband's shoulders—use imagination and creativity.)

## 8. PROPS

In the chapter on setting moods, we explored the utilization of props, from candles to showers to pillows. These positions use the furniture around your house as props as you increase your erotic playing together.

*Sitting on a chair.* The husband sits up straight on a chair that allows the wife to sit in his lap facing and straddling him. The penis is inserted with mutual effort. It is helpful if the wife's feet touch the floor or are propped up on pillows to ease insertion and to help create movement. This position, like other face-to-face positions, allows visual contact and kissing and holding and whispering or breathing in ears. The hands are free so the husband can caress back and buttocks. He may try cradling her buttocks in his hands to help produce movement with his arms. A variant of this position is to have the wife turn around and face away. Again, it is helpful if her feet can touch the floor. The husband can stroke breasts and clitoris while she reaches down and stimulates his penis with her fingers.

This position, like some of the other sitting positions, does not allow a great deal of thrusting motion. It can be quietly erotic; the connecting of intercourse does not always have to lead to rapid movement or produce a climax. Sitting positions can be playful, and they add variety.

*Wife on the edge.* The bed is a comfortable object for the wife to be on the edge of, but don't limit creativity. Dining

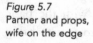
Figure 5.7
Partner and props,
wife on the edge

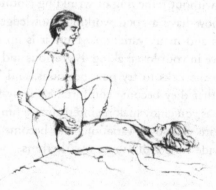

room tables, kitchen counters, couches, and easy chairs work well too.

The wife is positioned at the edge of the bed, sofa, or table. Her legs are around her husband's torso, resting comfortably on his thighs, with his arms supporting and clamping them to his body. The husband kneels or stands depending on the height of the object the wife is on, so his penis is accessible to her vagina. He has an easy thrusting motion, and the wife may not be fully reclined but propped up on the pillows of an easy chair and have access to stroking and caressing herself and her husband.

This position is very visually stimulating to the husband: he can observe the vulval area and the penis thrusting in and out. It is exciting to the wife: she can observe her partner's arousal by her body as well as experience her own visual excitement. Her vagina and clitoris receive excellent friction in this position. The wife-on-the-edge position works well during later stages of pregnancy or when the fatigued wife wants her husband to take the active role. It lends itself to all rooms of the house and provides some fun variation because it can be enjoyed without removing or wrinkling clothing.

You now have a good working knowledge with the basic positions and many variations. Now it is up to you to bring them alive in your lovemaking. Be curious and experimental as you take the risks to try new positions, and learn them well enough that they become comfortable. Truly frolic and laugh and love as you enjoy making intercourse a fun part of your sex life. Create your own variations and become lovingly at ease with a wide variety of moves and rhythms.

# 6

# MINIMIZING THE MESS

*W*hen contemplating marriage and their sex life to come, most couples don't think of "messy." The word *mess* is defined as "an untidy or unpleasant state." It certainly does fit many aspects of sex. It is unfortunate, but many couples let the mess seriously dampen their lovemaking. Minimizing the mess and controlling the environment are integral parts of making love. You can learn to live comfortably with untidiness, or you can let God's wonderful gift of sex be sabotaged. You will discover that what you thought was gross can be minimized or may actually become a fun part of mutual lovemaking.

## PHYSICAL SEXUALITY

A fundamental part of making love is that it is passionate, with physical arousal, active loveplay, and noise. One wife complained about how "animalistic" sex seemed to her. If you are an emotional person who can go down a waterslide with your mouth wide open screaming, the passionate part of sex won't seem that messy. If you enjoy sports and perspiring and don't worry about making a face and grunting when you hit a tennis ball, you probably won't be put off by the sheer physicalness of making love on a summer afternoon.

But you may not like to sweat or get too involved in feelings. You may have to give yourself permission to be erotically physical as you allow this activity to grow into being more romantic. Being wildly abandoned as you revel in your body and the body of your mate can seem very untidy and uncontrolled. To be a great lover, you will have to be open to becoming passionate and be adaptable to change as you learn to enjoy new and exciting experiences.

You'll make funny noises and unsettling mistakes as you enjoy making love. At some point the husband may miscalculate his time of ejaculation. Or his vocal excitement may render his wife nearly deaf if his mouth is too close to her ear. Or the wife may dribble evidence of her husband's recently spent passion when she sits astride his body. If you don't have a sense of humor or can't forgive yourself and your mate, sex won't be very much fun. Being sensual, passionate, and playful is never neat. Bodies and their functions are never totally romantic, but they can create some marvelous sexual connection.

It won't happen overnight, but active thrusting, sweat, semen, and vaginal secretions will become arousing stimulants of pleasure and sexual excitement as you associate them with your mate and fun times together. You and your mate can be open to each other's feelings. And you both can make an effort to anticipate when the other may consider seepage of the body's natural fluids to be unpleasant. The love you have for each other encourages you to control various activities so that enjoyment is equal. A box of tissues is a smart thing to keep around your bed anyway, to help you minimize the mess. Making love will slowly cease to seem as messy or out of control as you take steps to minimize the interferences and slowly change some attitudes.

## MENSTRUAL CYCLE

What is a good rule of thumb for lovemaking when the wife is in her menstrual cycle? Like other types of sexual interaction, it depends on the sensibilities of the individual and couple. Please sort through this situation carefully. Many couples lose some opportune times for making love by completely avoiding intercourse or other loveplay during this time. Here are some commonsense ideas you will need to discuss together as sexual lovers and partners:

1. There is nothing dirty about the menstrual flow, and there is nothing wrong with having sex during this time if a couple wishes. Both mates may have negative attitudes they need to talk through and resolve.

2. The vagina and genitals can be tender during menstruation, and during the heavy flow, many men and women prefer not to have intercourse. That does not negate making love—which you never want to associate solely with intercourse. There can still be mutual pleasuring through to orgasm and fun sex play. Because of aesthetics or tenderness, you may wish to avoid the days of heavy flow, however.

3. Though not foolproof, during and immediately after are safe times to have sex with a very low risk of pregnancy. Many couples enjoy sex during the lighter flow at the end of the period. They may put a towel under themselves and keep tissues

or a washcloth handy for cleanup afterward. Some couples find it enjoyable to have intercourse regardless of flow and take a quick shower after or even make love in the shower. It depends on your and your mate's sensitivities.

If you have not taken the time to talk through this aspect of minimizing the mess, do it now. You may assume you know what your mate thinks and feels, but your assumptions could get you in trouble and rob you of many permitted pleasures. Let the wife tell of her growing-up experiences and how she felt about her period over her developmental years. How do each of you feel aesthetically, and what would you feel comfortable trying sexually, during the menstrual cycle? Talk it through and come to some mutual understandings.

## BIRTH CONTROL

The Genesis passage on being fruitful and multiplying is in the context of God's giving humankind control of the natural world. We are to be wise stewards of the children God places in our care. To choose to have one or two or five has to be a thoughtful and prayerful decision.

You as a couple will have to sort through which method best fits you as you consider personal sensitivities and values, nuisance, health, and who takes responsibility. Some of you may come from a Catholic background and will have to sort through this whole concept. It is good for all of us to remember that God values family and procreation with the planting of seed and the possibility of conception.

I have abbreviated this section knowing that you can get

more information as needed, but what follows are the common methods of birth control. Obviously, none of these methods will be effective *unless carefully followed*. Birth control can either dump on your sex life or be managed gracefully.

## TYPES OF BIRTH CONTROL

*Rhythm or natural method*. This method is based on the fact that pregnancy occurs during ovulation when the sperm meets the egg. If you are trying to keep from getting pregnant, you will not want to have intercourse during the time of ovulation. Sperm live approximately two days and the female egg one day unless fertilized. Three methods are used to predict ovulation and gauge a "safe" period of time for intercourse. The first uses the calendar and considers that ovulation occurs around fourteen days before the onset of the menstrual flow. The second way of determining ovulation is through the woman's charting her temperature upon awakening. The third method involves observing the cervical mucus and learning the natural changes in its consistency around ovulation. The rhythm method poses no health risk and does not include apparatuses to dampen spontaneity. It does put a damper on intercourse during a significant part of the month.

*Contraceptive pill*. Birth control pills contain the synthetic hormone *estrogen* or *progestin* or a combination of the two. The pills alter the body's hormone balance and (a) prevent the ovaries from ovulating, (b) change the consistency of the cervical mucus, and (c) change the consistency of the fallopian tubes and the uterus. An advantage of the pill is that it does not interfere with naturalness. A couple can make love as the mood strikes. The pill, if properly used, has a high success rate of preventing pregnancy, although nothing is foolproof. It also can have side effects of weight gain and even dampening of sexual desire, so keep consulting with your physician.

*Condom.* Condom use is a method of birth control that the husband can take responsibility for. Here are some important instructions:

- Put the condom on before approaching the vagina, and be careful not to get seepage on the outside of the condom.
- Use a new condom for every ejaculation or act of inter-course—this prevents seepage or breakage with sperm in the condom.
- Withdraw the penis before the erection is fully lost, and above all, hold the condom as you withdraw the penis to prevent its slipping off.

An advantage of condoms is that they are easily available and effective if properly used, perhaps in conjunction with a spermicidal jelly. A disadvantage is that some men and women dislike the reduced sensation in the penis or the vagina. Condoms and other methods of birth control such as a diaphragm can be incorporated into the act of lovemaking. The wife can help create a romantic mood by unrolling the condom on her husband's penis as part of the loveplay.

*Female condom.* Female condoms are not a new concept but have recently been brought back on the market. Like the male condom, they are made of a thin, strong latex and are a sheath. The female variety has a flexible ring at each end and is inserted into the vagina before intercourse. The rings keep it in place, and it creates a protective lining in the vagina that contains the penis and sperm. The instructions for the male condom apply also to the female condom. Any barrier method loses some of the spontaneity.

*Diaphragm and cervical cap.* A diaphragm and a cervical cap are round rubber devices with a covered metal rim. Each is inserted into the vagina with spermicidal jelly, foam, or suppository as a barrier against the sperm swimming into the cervix and uterus. The diaphragm is inserted into the vagina behind the pubic bone and holds the spermicide over the cervix. The cervical cap is a smaller version of the diaphragm and covers only the cervix. A diaphragm or a cap needs to be fitted and prescribed by a gynecologist. It's advantage, like the sponge, is that it is easy to use and can be inserted prior to making love.

*Spermicidal sponge.* Available over the counter, the spermicidal sponge is dampened with water before inserting it into the vagina. This action releases the spermicidal foam. The sponge acts as a barrier, and it has spermicide to counteract impregnation. Like any barrier method, it is still somewhat intrusive and has to be prepared for ahead of time.

*Intrauterine devices.* Some IUDs have caused infections in the uterus and must be used with caution. For some women, they are still effective when used under a physician's care. The intrauterine device is a small coil or loop inserted into the uterus. Once inserted, it can be left in place for a year or more. It works by causing the uterus to reject the fertilized egg. For some couples, this might violate personal ethics. The IUD is long-term and effective and does not have the mess of the barrier methods.

*Spermicidal foam, jelly, and suppository.* These chemicals are inserted into the vagina and kill the sperm. Some women have to experiment to find ones that don't cause an allergic reaction. The spermicides can be used alone as a method of birth control, but this is not recommended. They are much more effective if used with a condom or a diaphragm.

*Note: Many failures of any method of birth control are due to the improper and careless application of that method.* This is not something you can afford to get sloppy or take chances with. Pray that God will help you to be wise, careful, and disciplined in this area of your life. It's a necessary part of lovemaking, and you can learn to gracefully adjust.

## TYPES OF LUBRICATION

In response to thrusting and other stimulation, our bodies produce lubrication to prepare for intercourse. The fact of the matter is that this will not always be adequate even if you are young and healthy. You may wish to stimulate sensitive tissues as a part of arousal, or you may be taking a decongestant that is making you dry, or prolonged lovemaking may need something extra. Every couple should have some artificial lubrication handy to use as needed as an aid to great lovemaking.

Many drugstores sell a variety of artificial lubricants in the same section as the condoms and spermicides. Vaseline is an old standby, but because it is not water-soluble, it can be more difficult for the vagina to be self-cleansing and for cleanup in general. K-Y Jelly is another standby that works well. Some couples complain that K-Y dries out, and they prefer a different type such as Astroglide or Wet. These are more liquid and come in small plastic dispensers. Wet also makes its Fun Flavors lubricants that taste good if oral stimulation is going to be enjoyed.

Many couples find natural oils from coconut to olive oil appealing for smell and consistency. They are edible and don't interfere with oral stimulation of the genitals. Vegetable oils (corn or safflower) work fine if you have forgotten to get something you like better. Take some time to experiment and find out what works best for you.

## MINIMIZING BIRTH CONTROL AND LUBRICATION

A theme of this chapter is minimizing the messy or needed but nuisance parts of sex. However, even better than minimizing the mess is taking these untidy aspects of sex and incorporating them in such a way that they enhance your lovemaking. You as lovers can make birth control and lubrication easier and more erotic.

Keep supplies readily available and easy to put into action. Getting up from bed and going to get them, not having them handy, or forgetting to purchase them put a damper on spontaneity. Incorporate them into your loveplay and erotic arousal. Putting on the condom or inserting the diaphragm can be very stimulating. Lubrication can be slowly and sensuously applied.

Both of you should take responsibility for birth control and lubrication. Don't make it the sole job of either mate. Share in the purchase and use of whatever method you choose. Stay creative and keep a fun variety. Try different kinds of lubrication. Sometimes don't include intercourse so you don't have to deal with birth control if you are using a barrier method. Keep as spontaneous, playful, and sensuous as you can. Consider these key qualities you need in dealing with the messiness of a great sex life:

- *Sense of humor.* Laughing together and not taking yourself so seriously are invaluable. Sex will be funny and full of mishaps and playfulness.

- *Flexibility.* Keep out of routines and let go of a strong need to always be in control. You will enjoy yourself more in making love if you can go with the flow and are able to adapt.

- *Forgiveness.* Let each other make mistakes, and let go of resentment and hurt. Allow each other to change as both work through tough areas, and cut each other some slack as both focus on positive solutions. Forgiveness is the cleansing agent that makes for great marriages and great sex lives.

- *Effective communication.* A couple must be able to assertively express needs and feelings and truly hear each other. No topic is off-limits, and with dialogue and compromise, solutions can be reached.

- *Love and trust.* If you like each other and believe your mate wants you to be happy and sexually fulfilled, it is easier to discuss and negotiate. An intimate relationship is vital in responsibly using birth control, creatively experimenting, and flexibly communicating.

- *Being disciplined.* This trait may seem in direct contrast to the final point, but minimizing the mess requires both. A couple must carefully follow the prescribed birth control's directions. Remembering ahead to have tissues or lubricants can make a real difference in spontaneity.

- *Being uninhibited.* Let yourself go as you enjoy your mate and God's gift of sex. Being uninhibited and sensual has a way of overcoming and transforming the muss of sex into an aphrodisiac.

You and your partner can ensure that the untidiness of sex never gets in the way of a thriving love life. Let God give you the wisdom to find those many creative compromises and solutions.

# 7

# Sexual Communication

$\mathcal{D}$o you want to fall deeper in love and create a truly passionate marriage? Effective communication is at the heart of this process. Becoming more passionate means letting down your walls as you create the safety and trust to really talk about sex and become lovers. Strive for a "naked and unashamed" ability to let each other into your most private places. I am amazed by how many partners in solid marriages are not able to discuss sexual concerns or desires—forfeiting this deeper level of connection and passion.

The following questions illustrate the courage and openness needed to engage in sexual conversations: Who will initiate sex the most? What would be your ideal sexual experience? Will you want sex during your period? What does oral sex mean to you? Will you be willing to experiment with new behaviors such as positions of intercourse? Risk the tough issues. Open and honest communication builds an intimate, fulfilling companionship, which is the catalyst for great sex. The more you communicate about sex and your love life, the more passionately you will love and become that awesome lover.

# EMPATHY: THE KEY TO GREAT COMMUNICATION

The essence of effective communication is a dialogue that ends in empathy. One partner has assertively stated his or her reality, and the other partner has been able to walk in his or her shoes to understand and acknowledge that reality. This is what empathy is all about—understanding. It is not agreeing. Mature communicators in this dialogue process abandon the need to *win, debate, convince,* or *make a point.* One partner talks while the other truly listens and works through to empathy.

*Assertively **state** your personal reality.* Start with "I" statements that take responsibility without blaming (not "*You* turn me off," but "*I* feel my desire shut down when you grab at me"). Assertive communication is direct and respectful without being aggressive or passive. Risk conflict and express your core feelings and needs (not "*You're* a lousy lover," but "*I* need you to remember to initiate; it makes me feel desired").

*Objectively **empathize** with your partner's reality.* Express understanding of your partner's message with short empathy summaries. Remember, empathy is not agreeing that your mate's reality is free of distortions or accepting their feelings as correct and true; instead, it is going beyond the surface content to acknowledge the deeper needs and feelings.

Take the questions addressed above and talk them through with one expressing their opinions and feelings while the other partner listens and empathizes. Empathy summaries might start with: "That makes sense to me that you . . . ," or "You must feel . . . ," "I can understand how . . . ," or "You're need-ing me to . . ." (not "You shouldn't feel that way," but "I can understand how you could feel embarrassed and uncomfort-able having sex during your period"). Switch roles of assertively stating realities after the partner who is conveying his or her reality agrees that the other has understood and that the empathy statements are accurate. Empathy skills are espe-cially crucial in resolving sexual conflicts.

*Learn to manage emotionally-loaded topics in the partner-ship.* There are skills that great communicators utilize to keep negotiating and conflict resolution clean and productive. Sexual disagreements can stem from very different needs and expectations.

- Stick to the topic.
- Pick your battles and develop your timing.
- Remain courteous.
- Set limits (stop when it becomes irrational or late at night).
- Reconcile the relationship (forgive, apologize, emphasize your love).

I cannot stress enough the importance of communication skills in working through sexuality in dating, on the honey-moon, and in the years to come. Continue to improve your nonsexual communication so you are even better at your sex-ual communication. Read a book (a great one is *A Lasting Promise: A Christian Guide to Fighting for Your Marriage* by Stanley, Trathen, McCain & Bryan [San Francisco: Jossey-Bass, 1998]), watch a video, or listen to an audiotape together on improving communication in your marriage. Talk about what tips and techniques you would like to try to implement in your couple communication.

## THE LANGUAGE OF LOVEMAKING

Sex is a difficult, private topic. Couples can often make love more easily than they can talk about it. Assertively discussing what they need does not come easily for many people, especially in the sexual arena. Erotic communication must be developed.

### VOCABULARY AND SLANG

In developing a sexual vocabulary, you may be wondering if slang is ever appropriate. Of course, slang is permissible and fun and erotic. Your pet names for body parts and secret vocabulary shared by only the two of you contain a lot of slang and euphemisms. As a couple you will find various words expressive and arousing. As Christians, however, we must be careful to avoid the very negative attitudes and ideas about sex that society over the centuries has incorporated into slang. We never want to be foolish, aggressive, or demeaning.

Learn to converse openly about making love without shame or embarrassment, and talk during sex. Expand your vocabulary, and adapt slang that both of you enjoy for body parts and activities. I laugh in counseling sessions, and it doesn't take much imagination to understand when clients talk about "Big John" or "Shamu" wanting to "dive into your pool, but you fell asleep." Sex is your playground, and great communication means fun.

## NONVERBAL SIGNALS

Build up a fun and useful repertoire of nonverbal language. Experts speculate that anywhere from 65 to 95 percent of communication is nonverbal, so it is no wonder that great lovers master this aspect of connecting. Try not to mind-read or assume; check out or establish some of the nonverbal signals verbally. Perhaps gentle pressure with a hand signals the desire to shift into another position. Groans, sighs, and exclamations may signal degrees of arousal and when to proceed to another phase of lovemaking. (Warning: Do practice a little discretion when visiting your parents.) A certain outfit or lack thereof may be a signal of sexual availability. Nonverbal communication helps orchestrate a sex life that will grow ever more comfortable and meaningful.

Develop nonverbal signals that indicate your desire for sexual activity. Without allowing it to completely lose its subtlety, make sure the nonverbal vocabulary is accurate and obvious enough. It may be a passionate hug or kiss. Sometimes an amorous look or a soft kiss on the back of the neck is all it takes.

## LOVE TALK

How much do you talk before sex? During sex? After sex? Talking really is a great way to enhance your sex life. Each of these three areas of erotic communication—before, during, and after making love—has its unique excitement and sexual stimulation.

1. *Love talk before.* One couple related how their fun lovemaking was built on phone calls during the day that created anticipation and arousal. Another told of their E-mails that they tried to be sure to delete. Wives often state that they do not keep

sex on the front burner as their husbands do, but that this kind of communication creates fantasies and desire. They enjoy approaches that are teasing but do not lead to immediate sex.

Everyone loves surprises. The wife who tells her husband on the way into the party that she is not wearing panties and can't wait till later that evening will certainly enhance their future activity. The husband tenderly telling his wife how sexy she is before falling asleep on a Friday night is engaging in some great pre-lovemaking communication. Unleash your creativity with this great aphrodisiac.

2. *Love talk during.* During sex, the idea is to relax and let the talk be free-flowing on what you are feeling and sensing. Sometimes you and your mate will be on a common theme, and at other times each will pursue personal images—both can be connecting and stimulating sexually. The wife might say, "You sure are hitting the right spot inside me." And the husband might reply, "You feel so good, I wish I could do this all night." Or the husband might go off on his own tangent: "I'm glad you're feeling excited. That dance you did to seduce me tonight was unbelievable."

During making love, you can also tease and talk about fantasies. This talk can be very erotic as both get into creating the mood. Tell your partner what you want and need sexually in a given session. If something pops into your mind that you two haven't tried in a while, bring it up and both may enter into the activity with gusto. Erotic communication has so much potential.

3. *Love talk after.* This should be a time of talking and warm reminiscing, of talking and reaffirming your love for each other, of talking and appreciating how truly close you two have

become. You are perhaps closest to the Garden of Eden at this time in your intimate connection. Like Adam and Eve, during your lovemaking you have become naked without any shame.

It's a different kind of love talk, but it's so bonding. Don't neglect this afterglow time of nonverbal and verbal linking. Even a simple "You mean so much to me" takes on special significance during this vulnerable, united time. Mates especially feel vulnerable and need this affirmation because they have both physically and emotionally opened themselves up to each other.

## COACHING

A wife may think her husband is supposed to know all about sex. Or a couple may wonder why they are the only couple in the world whose sex life has not automatically fallen into place. After all, if making love is supposed to be such a natural thing, why are they struggling? The truth is, like marriage in general, two unique male and female persons getting together will have differences. No matter how technically skilled they are, their sexual relationship will be a blending of two unique bodies and varying attitudes and needs.

Coaching is all about assertively expressing your sexual needs and feelings, learning to problem-solve around difficult areas, and helping your mate understand you. This section considers three areas of making love that will need some coaching.

### INITIATING AND REFUSING

All successful lovers have to polish their skills in initiating and refusing. No couple is immune from some misunderstandings in this area of sexual communication and attitudes.

Think for a moment about what is at stake that makes initiating and refusing become so symbolic and filled with disappointments and hurt feelings. First, initiating and refusing make one vulnerable to rejection and feelings of abandonment. Second, ineffective initiating attempts can make a person feel pushed, controlled, and treated like a sexual object. Third, much of initiating is nonverbal and therefore open to misinterpretation. Fourth, initiating, or the lack thereof, becomes synonymous with sexual desire and sexual appeal. Fifth, initiating or refusing sex means coordinating two unique people with different needs and priorities on a given day or hour.

It's understandable why this is a loaded topic that must be discussed with both partners open to coaching! Great lovers take the time and energy to understand their mates, learn required skills, and make needed changes as they initiate and refuse effectively.

## MAXIMIZING

In your sex life there are some things your mate does that really turn you on and others that really turn you off. You have to tell your partner what you want and what you dislike, including specific behaviors and attitudes that are appreciated or get in the way. You want to maximize your sex life? Talk! Coach! Emphasize and practice the positive!

Here are some important guidelines for giving helpful suggestions as you coach your mate and maximize your sex life:

1. Major coaching should be done fully clothed as you dialogue about your sex life. Subjects could be poor hygiene,

inhibitions, boredom, pushiness, and/or technique deficits. Stay humble and self-confident as you listen to criticism. Allow yourself to be in a nondefensive mode as you create skills for a lifetime partnership.

2. Minor adjusting needs comfortable nonverbal (touches and noises) and verbal language that can be done nonthreateningly. For example, you might say, "That hurts," "Slow down," "You're on my arm," "More," "Shift."

3. Know thyself! Acquire wisdom! It is tough coaching if you are not sure what you need or want. Read, experiment, give yourself permission to be uninhibitedly sexual as you become truly self-aware. Great coaches know and utilize the player's abilities.

4. Focus on the positive! The primary goal of coaching is to maximize strengths and bring out the best in players—not correct what's wrong. Great coaching employs many methods: demonstrate by doing it on yourself or guiding your mate's hand, talk and exchange data, buy books and use them as your assistant coaches, go to a sex therapist, and start with small changes.

## ROADBLOCKS

Quite often a couple feels that they are the only ones whose sex life isn't easy and effortless. However, many newlyweds experience some kind of sexual difficulty. It may be a lack of desire, temporary impotence, conflict around frequency, an inability to let go of control, problems reaching a climax, or old wounds.

All the things you have already read about sexual communication especially apply to roadblocks. You can't sweep them under the rug because they won't go away. They can be embarrassing to discuss, and they are emotionally loaded. Communication skills really count now. Choose a setting where there is plenty of time and privacy. Keep clarifying the message as you focus and really try to understand your mate's needs and feelings. Detach from your anger and fear as you listen and empathize with your partner's assertive sharing of what is happening. Truly walk in each other's shoes.

You may need some professional help, but first read an appropriate chapter in a book and start talking. Sexual communication has some marvelous healing capacities. A central part of most sexual difficulties is anxiety (fears, worry, guilt) or anger (irritation, disappointment, disrespect, hostility). Talking about the difficulty and acknowledging its impact keep lovers from being so anxious and avoiding sex.

Anger and disappointment can quickly distance lovers as hurt and disrespect grow. It is painful and tough at times, but there is no substitute for talking through the problem. Talking defuses the tension, creates understanding and acceptance, and promotes changes. Yes, it may take professional assistance from a sex or marital therapist, but start your own honest, open dialogue.

Husbands and wives, especially husbands, need to take responsibility to learn effective communication skills. Develop a great sexual vocabulary, and enjoy erotic communication. Talk before, during, and after you make love as you enhance the entire experience. God has given you a wonderful aphrodisiac in your ability to communicate!

## TIME OUT . . .

1. Make love this week, and agree ahead of time that you will make noise—exaggerate and enjoy it. Keep up a running commentary on what you are feeling and sensing. Nonverbal communication can be tremendously exciting.

2. Practice this assignment frequently: Fully clothed, sit and discuss what modifications you would like to make in your sex life. Be specific, and explain what you wish your mate would do more and less of. Arrange a time for a lovemaking session in which you institute and practice one mate's suggestions and a separate time for the other's suggestions. Be sure to use the four ideas for maximizing your sex life.

## 8

# MAKING LOVE TO YOUR WIFE

*M*en desperately want to be competent at all they do. Making love can seem a real setup because your wife will often be a deep mystery to you. Women are so beautifully complex. You think you know a lot and you're trying to be a great lover, but then you hit another bump in the road. Let's try to understand some of this mystery so that making love to your wife can become more exciting and less frustrating for both of you.

## UNIQUELY FEMALE

Begin this journey by trying to walk in your wife's moccasins as you grow in understanding and skills. There is a uniqueness to her that is helpful to know.

### WARMLY CONNECTED SOUL MATES

In the wise, biblical way of "becoming one flesh," women can't divorce sex as easily from the relational and emotional aspects as men can. A woman wants to feel cared about and emotionally connected before sexual activity can have appeal. For her, fun sex flows out of an intimate companionship that is emotionally close with plenty of physical affection and quality time together. *Conveying this attitude and these feelings is not something you can do quickly in the hour before you want sex.* Intimate connecting involves daily and hourly choices. Pay attention to her: give her two compliments every day, tell her things you notice and appreciate about her, come out of your cave and talk more.

Your tenderness and attentiveness may be more erotic to your wife than great techniques. Doing the dishes, calling her during the day, or tenderly listening can be a sexual turn-on—if she knows you are doing this from the heart and not for the purpose of getting sex. Time spent in loveplay draws her closer than time spent producing orgasms. The different paths to the souls of men and women could be charted as follows:

MEN: Physical activity → connects the soul → leads to emotional closeness.

WOMEN: Emotional closeness → connects the soul → opens the door to physical activity.

## VIVE LA ROMANCE

People are not born romantic. Romance is a combination of skills and attitudes that are learned. What is this romance that women yearn for and need to have included in their sex lives and relationships? The words *"special sweetheart"* describe the attitude your wife desires from you. Your passionate focus on her as if she is the only woman in the world makes her feel special.

Women are certainly on target in demanding romance as a necessary component of making love. *Vive la romance!* Great sex does indeed originate from your imaginative creativity and those mushy cards, erotic candlelit bedrooms, sexy dates, and holding hands.

## CONSISTENTLY INCONSISTENT

You may wonder why your wife is physically inconsistent. On one evening she may like oral arousal or enjoy her breasts and nipples being caressed, and at another time she may not want that particular stimulation at all. Her body and reactions do not stay consistent, and you get confused. The fact is, she does change in what is arousing to her. Sometimes her clitoris is more sensitive than at other times, and a particular stroke is more irritating than exciting. A firm, rapid stroke might feel good later on in a lovemaking session but is annoying for her initially. Your penis is very consistent, and most times it responds to firm stimulation. But your wife's body does not function in this way.

Develop a series of strategies for making love. Become adept at smoothly switching gears, from strategy A to strategy B to strategy E, depending on where your wife is in a given lovemaking session. Encourage her to say what she wants. Sometimes she may just want to nurture you, and you may climax as quickly as you want to. At other times she may desire gentle massage of nonerogenous zones or her breasts. Expect inconsistency and revel in your fast footwork and improvisational skills. Become a skilled lover as you vary approaches and rhythms and types of stimulation. She will love your spontaneous variety.

Your wife may not have the same consistent type of desire that you do. This may be hormonal, and you can enjoy certain times in her menstrual cycle. The inconsistency may also be relational and environmental, and you can help make changes to alleviate stress and create romance. Your desires are just different in what you find stimulating and arousing—in what turns you on and turns you off. Talk about it and negotiate.

## VULNERABLE TO DISTRACTION

Husbands can falsely assume that their wives don't like sex as much as they do. They don't understand that their wives are more easily distracted by their environment and their inner attitudes and feelings. When she is fatigued, struggling with body image, feeling hurt, or in the bedroom next to her mom's, she may be unable to focus on sex and her desire to make love will be on the back burner.

Your wife, more than you, may have to fight distractions during actual lovemaking as she focuses on her own arousal. The wise husband minimizes distractions (e.g., the bedroom is picked up, phone calls have been made) and helps his wife begin to make love (romantic suggestion when leaving for work, sexy kissing in living room when he comes home) even before they are in the bedroom. Be sensitive to her concerns. You are less susceptible to distractions and often want to make love without the mood having to be exactly right. As you are more supportive and involved, she may be in the mood more often. Your wife will find making love more appealing and restorative as the distractions are acknowledged and controlled.

## MAKING LOVE AN EMOTIONAL
## CHOICE WITH A WARM-UP TIME

Your wife is more likely to make a cognitive decision when she wants to make love and appreciates having the opportunity to create the right mental and emotional attitude. It isn't the more immediate, hormonal surge that it can be with you. Wives love surprises and being spontaneous, but they are usually not crazy about quickies or jumping into bed the minute the vacation destination is reached. Sex is more purposeful, romantic, and intimate with a woman. She will not think of sex as often as you do and this is not lack of desire. *You can learn a lot from each other* with her emotional decision (sometimes this decision is made when you initiate) to nurture and be with you, and your impulsive readiness to jump right in.

Your wife has to want sex and choose to make love in ways that are consistent with how she is feeling, with emotional and affectional attachment. The timing must be appropriate with plenty of loveplay as her body and emotions are "primed" and she is allowed to choose to respond in her own passionate way. Women often take fifteen to twenty minutes to reach an orgasm. This is partly physical and partly because she needs time to overcome distractions as she mentally and emotionally allows arousal. You were ready when she took her shirt off, but she will take more time. When lovemaking occurs and she is willingly involved, she can respond with receptive desire and a passionate enjoyment that will surprise you.

## GENTLE AND TEASING AND SLOW— THEN VIGOROUS

Wives often complain that their husbands are too direct, speedy, or entirely too predictable. Men often have a real skill deficit in the art of touching softly, approaching gently, and keeping a teasing variety in lovemaking. There can be too much pawing and grabbing and going for the goodies.

Especially in initial loveplay, women often prefer gentle, teasing caresses, and may like intercourse to start off with easy, shallow thrusts. She may like to flirt and start making love with clothes still on. She may love it when you tease her body and softly blow in her ear, kiss her neck, and do not immediately head for her breasts or genitals. The pleasure will gradually grow and will be exciting when you take the time to playfully torment her by coming on then backing off.

*Slow* is the operative word in fantastic sex. Teasing arousal by its very nature takes time, but a gradual, unhurried, leisurely pace will be greatly appreciated by your mate. Often she will take longer to reach arousal, and this will allow her that time to enter into the lovemaking fully.

As you follow her lead, your wife depends on you to create the rhythm of your lovemaking. She will not always want it slow and soft. As she becomes aroused the pace can get vigorous and fast. Then you can think of what feels good to you and duplicate it with her. She will want stronger stimulation of the clitoral area and intercourse can be a wilder experience. Genital pleasuring can become the focus and orgasm is now more the intent.

## MULTIPLE ORGASMS

Women are multi-orgasmic; men are not. A woman can have a series of orgasms, one right after the other. Men have a recuperative time between orgasms that can increase from minutes to hours with age. Some wives may experience two or more separate orgasms in a couple of minutes with a short pause or rest between each.

But don't get hung up on numbers or multiple orgasms! Help your wife enjoy her orgasmic potential, but let go of any need to create more or deeper climaxes. She won't be keeping score as long as you are growing in your lovemaking skills. The intensity and number of orgasms will follow and will vary from session to session of lovemaking.

## EROTIC SYMBOLISM AND SENSUALITY

What do women find sexy in men? Gentle or sexy or attentive looks are turn-ons. Stomachs and buttocks that are kept in shape are often on the list, along with grooming in general. Talking and being vulnerable are important; the ability to express feelings is very attractive and arouses erotic feelings. Minds are often considered sexy, and men are pleasing who can be passionate about life or a cause. Wives are excited by their husbands' ability to take charge but not be controlling. They want a skilled lover who can take them into passion assertively.

Your wife may enjoy smells and sounds and touch in ways you never thought to appreciate. Silk or satin negligees, warm lotion, fragrant flowers, or rollicking jazz enhance the experience. Making love can become more interesting and arousing as you learn from her sensual temperament and incorporate a wider range of erotically stimulating symbols. Don't get hung up on what you think is sexy and sensual, but instead learn from her. Peach-colored satin draped sexily over a breast may be more sensuous than the black-lace cutout you had in mind.

## FOR MEN ONLY

Men can shoot themselves in the foot on their way to becoming the world's greatest lover. In this section, we will consider how easy it is for men to miss the mark and sacrifice quality sexual bonding. We need to truly love our wives with passion, wisdom, and depth.

### 3-D WOMEN

Men have a difficult time letting women be three-dimensional, with body, soul, and spirit. The preoccupation with the body aspect of sex actually puts a damper on the true fun God intended. Husbands who learn to notice and make love to the total person create an awesome passion with a deeper sexual connecting. Practice 3-D sex and quit being one-dimensional.

*Body.* Observe her eyes, which are the windows to the soul—is she happy, sad, tired, excited? Look at less common but very feminine body parts like earlobes, hands, mouth, and posture.

*Soul.* Be aware of emotions—what is her style of enjoying life and people? Observe her mind and heart—know that she needs attention and affirmation, not lust.

*Spirit.* Know she wants someone special in her life to adore and cherish. Think of her need for intimate connecting. Has she allowed God to meet her deep inner desires too?

### MALE MYTHOLOGY

Probably the most prevalent male myth concerns the size of the penis. Do some self-talk and get over any feeling of inferiority. It's not the size that counts but how you enjoy sensuality and use it. Remember the old saying: "It's not the size of the boat, but the motion of the ocean."

Along with the size-of-penis myth is the idea that a woman is turned on by hard, deep thrusting in intercourse. Your wife will enjoy and be more turned on by softer, smoother, and at times more rapid, motions in intercourse as you make love to her tender genitals. A variant of this myth is that a really sexy wife will want her husband to take her immediately and then will go into fits of ecstasy as his penis fills her vagina.

Another devastating myth is that men know all about sex and are always ready to go sexually. We have our knowledge and desire deficits just like women, but we often feel guilty admitting them. All of us, as lovers, feel very deficient and inhibited at times as well as just plain worn out.

*Start letting go of your myths.* Your wife is probably quite average in desire, and you don't have to be a sexual machine. Don't assume that problems are all hers or yours. Look at ways that you both might be contributing to a lack of sexual frequency and other concerns you have in your lovemaking.

## MACHO SENSITIVITY

Your wife will be able to blossom as a woman and as a lover as you are able to sensitively understand and affirm her. You may need to start with affirming yourself and your body image and sexual self-esteem. Accept the size of your penis, trust your ability to acquire whatever skills you need to be an adept lover, and exercise your romantic creativity. Here are some ideas to practice that can help you be a sensitive, focused lover:

*Get a Ph.D in "My Wife."* Listen to her, observe her, increase your attention span, ask questions, try different things as you collect data, and be willing to make changes to please her. Husbands, your wives' femininity is precious and unique. Take the time to read a great book called *Secrets of Eve* (Hart, Weber & Taylor, Word 1998) and learn more of how she is wired sexually and what it will take to make her truly flourish. She will get turned on that you care enough to read a book about her. Unloading the dishwasher, or thoughtfully doing things to show her you care, will turn her on. Remember, it is not how hard you try but how smart you try. As much as you wish it, she will not respond like you, and you are going to have to learn some new skills.

*Gain a working knowledge of feelings.* It is especially important sexually that you learn to empathize and express excitement, dissatisfaction, gentleness, joy and happiness, contentment, discomfort, and pleasure.

*Cultivate softness, humility, gentleness, and love.* Learn to have a light touch and a soft, empathetic approach. Practice gentle responses and the strategy of going slow. Cultivate this feminine side of your masculine personality. It is a vital part of being a sensitive and adept lover—your wife will melt.

*Forget your obsessions.* You may have some fantasies you find sexy that she never will. She may never want to make love on an elevator or have oral sex on an airplane. You may also become obsessed with some part of her body that you wish were sexier. Do not and I repeat, do not, tell her this. Confess it to a buddy so he can tell you to grow up. Let go of your obsessions so you can enjoy the fullness of a great sex life and not shoot yourself in the foot.

## Passionate Leader

Most wives want husbands who are strong and confident and can provide unasked-for nurturing. They would like men who are not always predictable but have spontaneous energy and mystery. Wives at times want to be "taken"—not in a demanding or abusive way but out of a passionate desire for their femininity from a self-confident husband. They want to be swept off their feet and romantically enjoyed in wild and wonderful ways.

They also desire men who have sexual expertise but are able to implement suggestions without pouting and shutting down. They love men who are secure enough to appreciate and follow their lead at times too. Don't be predictable. Surprises bring a jolt of energy to the relationship as you increase your image of being mysterious, romantic, and passionate. She may think she has you figured out, but keep her off balance with impromptu romantic flourishes: come home early, massage her whole body with coconut butter, compliment her three times in one day. Mystery, variety, and strength are very sexy to your wife. Keep humble and secure and non-defensive as you evolve into a passionate leader.

## The Expert Lover

I am amazed at the number of wives in counseling who want their husbands to learn to kiss or include kissing more in their repertoire of lovemaking techniques. Guys, creative kissing can make your wife feel tremendously in love and alive.

## THE ART OF KISSING

Women enjoy variety in kissing, and the mouth can be extremely sensuous.

*Butterfly kisses.* Lightly kiss all over her face and body, keeping lips soft and gentle.

*Gently sucking.* Try this on your wife's nipple, her fingers or toes, her neck, or her lower lip.

*Warm, connecting kisses.* Plant a warm, juicy kiss on your wife's cheek or forehead as you walk by. It lets her know you enjoy her companionship and not just the sexual relationship.

*Deep kissing.* There is something passionate and intimate about sharing mouths and tongues. Don't fill her mouth with your tongue or shove it down her throat. Long, exciting kisses where you have to come up for breath should vary between playful tongue contact (don't immediately go beyond her teeth), warm and easy nibbling of her lower lip or earlobe, and deep, passionate sharing of tongues and souls. Breathe heavy and allow yourself to become aroused as you make kissing a drawn-out affair.

## MAKING LOVE TO HER BREASTS AND BODY

Breasts and nipples are very symbolic of femininity. They are erotically charged and an important part of the sexual anatomy to both you and your wife. Compliment, appreciate, admire, and enjoy them—don't grab, squeeze, or instantly rub.

Making love to your wife's breasts, like all of making love, should teasingly progress from light touches to more direct stimulation. Move in light, circular touches around the nipples or navel. Don't stop in one spot at first, but keep moving all over her body, briefly lingering on the more erogenous areas. This will progress to more direct and vigorous stimulation.

## PRIVATE INTIMACY

Part of the beauty and bonding nature of making love is choosing to allow another person, your special mate, into the most private areas of your life and body. Your wife allows you, her husband, to explore and enjoy her vulva, vagina, and clitoris in ways she has probably never even done herself. You need an intimate understanding of her body, especially her clitoris.

The clitoris is the central organ for stimulating sexual arousal in your mate. Expecting your wife to have an orgasm through vaginal stimulation alone (without carefully stimulating the clitoral area) is like her expecting you to climax by rubbing your testicles (without stimulating your penis). The clitoris is another part of the female anatomy that will need an indirect approach. Don't head for it immediately.

There are three positions of intercourse that your wife will find especially exciting because they enable you to provide direct manual stimulation to her clitoris: (1) the scissors position: you can take your erect penis and use it as a wand to stimulate her clitoris or you can use your fingers; (2) the husband in back in the spoon position: use your hand to caress buttocks, breasts, and tummy as well as inner thighs and clitoris; and (3) the wife-on-top position: leaves your thumb positioned to stimulate the clitoral area—women enjoy this position as they feel more in charge of their arousal and get great stimulation. (For details, see Chapter 5.)

God has given you a precious gift in creating for you your

own special woman and putting you into a one-flesh companionship with her. Together you two can enjoy excitement and intimacy! Maximize His gift as you courageously and wisely become a skilled and passionate leader and lover.

TIME OUT . . .

Men, pick out two ways you want to become a passionate leader for your wife. Really surprise her and discuss this with her so you can get her input and desires. We sometimes have difficulty setting our wives' needs as our priorities and truly following through—make sure you don't drop the ball with this one as you practice these leadership skills.

*9*

# MAKING LOVE TO YOUR HUSBAND

$\mathcal{M}$any times you have probably been amazed at the way your husband thinks and acts sexually. From the male perspective, there are few situations where sex doesn't add some spice and enhance the relationship. He can seem so one-track and grabby.

Making love is perhaps the primary means your husband uses to feel connected to you. He allows emotions to come out and himself to be physically close in a special way during your lovemaking. He also utilizes his sexual feelings to create variety and excitement in his life, perhaps letting sex have too prominent a place in his thinking and needs. As you read the following pages, you will discover he has a different sexual reality from yours. You may have to make some changes in the way you think, feel, and act to please him and improve your love life. But it is interesting that you are probably more similar sexually than you are different.

I must also state that some couples who are reading this book will find their situation reversed, with the wife having the stronger urge for lovemaking. Men can be overwhelmed and feel incompetent, have a lower desire, possess a fear of intimacy, or get their feelings hurt. The goal, regardless of which partner is more amorous, is to heal and negotiate and create a passionate and frequent sex life.

## UNIQUELY MALE

Are men different or simply more immature sexually than women? Some of your husband's actions and attitudes may stem from immaturity, with some needed changes being helpful. Much of his thinking and behavior, though, is due to the fact that you and he are wired differently. This section explains some of these distinctions.

### NO MENSTRUAL CYCLE, MORE APPARENT DESIRE

Female hormonal fluctuation is tied to the menstrual cycle. Obviously, men do not experience this cycle. The primary hormone in the male, testosterone, remains at a steady level within the male body until aging has some effects. Though this is not always true, many women find some of their sexual desire tied to the hormonal cycle while men do not experience this phenomenon. Their testosterone (the hormone that creates desire in both men and women) creates a fairly consistent desire.

That the male desire is apparently (more noticeable but not necessarily) stronger may also be a psychological as well as a biological occurrence. Because of the double standard in our society, boys are given a freer rein of their sexual curiosity and experimentation. They are encouraged to tune in to sex more as they, at an earlier age, build a strong, visual arousal to sexual cues.

Because men use making love as a primary way of connecting with their mates, their sexual desire can seem greater because the sexual part of the relationship may carry the load of maintaining intimacy. The need for more sexual activity can stem from an inability to connect in other ways, like conversations and nonsexual touching. But men are not sexual machines that are always switched on. They can be angry or stressed out or have defensive walls up that can sabotage their ability to relate sexually.

## VISUALLY SPECIFIC AND GENITALLY FOCUSED WITH MENTAL IMAGERY

You can't have helped seeing how your husband is prone to noticing parts of the female anatomy. Research has shown that both men and women are aroused by visual stimulation, but they have different styles. A woman can drive by a cute male jogger, notice his strong physique, and immediately forget the visual stimulus. A man can see a female jogger and almost drive off the road trying to see in the rearview mirror what her breasts are like. He is more specific and obvious in his pursuit of visual sexual cues. If he sees you in panties, he doesn't stop there. He mentally takes one cue and tunes in to other sexual cues almost reflexively in his fantasy life.

It is fun for men and women to help expand each other's mental imagery and use of fantasy. While the husband is tuning in to her bikini bottom and hidden genitals, the wife is noticing his gentle strength, feeling the soft breeze, and dreaming of making love in a secluded spot on the beach.

Men, in general, have to work harder to discipline their

thought life and tune out some of the sexual cues in the environment. They can more easily depersonalize sex as they tune in to erogenous zones more quickly than their wives do. That can lead to objectifying a woman, seeing her as a sexual object rather than as a total person. But there is a positive side to this trait.

Focusing visually on sexuality can also be exciting as your husband appreciates and affirms your femininity. His excitement and arousal can be contagious. You may find yourself tuning in to sexual cues more readily and learning from his openness to sexuality.

Great sex is built on going from general arousal to stimulating specific locations. You naturally tend to enjoy the general and teasing arousal, while he more enjoys the excitement of specific locations. It is fun to combine these different styles. You will find that a part of you enjoys a focus on erotic zones, and he can appreciate a more general, sensual approach. Each of you may find similarities you didn't know existed.

## IMMEDIATE AND QUICKER

Your husband has a tendency toward a more immediate sexual arousal and gratification with his visual specificity, genital focus, and mental imagery. You may enjoy an occasional spontaneous, quick encounter but not as much as he does. In the sexual cycle, you will take longer to reach an orgasm. He will climax more rapidly. This difference in quickness will require some accommodation.

Wives may sometimes wonder if their husbands have remained sexual adolescents (even though it adds zest to their lovemaking). He thinks about sex a lot; he tends to forget consequences and jump into pleasure, whether it means being late to a party or messing up her lipstick; he touches and grabs at what he likes; he loves the excitement of the moment, even if brief, and then savors these incidents to talk and think about later. He often has a short attention span sexually and will skip to something that seems to offer more fun. These qualities in your mate can be endearing, even though sometimes they drive you crazy.

## PREDICTABLE

What turns you on physically today might vary tomorrow. Sometimes you want direct clitoral stimulation, and sometimes you do not. But your husband is very predictable. If you appeal to him visually or rub his penis, he gets excited.

In some ways it can be fun that your husband is an easy read. When you take risks and initiate something silly or different, it will seldom flop. Try to remember to include visual stimuli, some immediate gratification, and friction on specific locations. You have a lot of power in a fun way sexually because he responds so predictably.

## TURNING YOURSELF ON

Every wife should be able to tune in to and enjoy the wonderful gift God has given her of femininity and a capacity for sexual pleasure. You may be wondering, in a chapter devoted to turning your husband on, why a whole section is now being devoted to turning yourself on. The answer is twofold: (1) Your husband is sexually excited by the sounds and sights of you tuning in to your own sexual pleasure and intensely enjoying the whole process. You want to turn him on and be a great lover? Learn to be intensely turned on yourself! (2) You face more hurdles in getting turned on and it helps to be self-aware as you appropriate God's unique gift of your feminine sexiness.

## PERMISSION FOR PLEASURE

God has given us a sexual celebration in marriage. The sad fact is that in Christianity, sex has often been feared and not talked about. Part of the distortion and confusion is created because of the silence as well as negative messages. Anyone becomes suspicious about a topic that is constantly avoided. You may have to erase mental tapes going around in your head from Mom or Dad, the church, and society to truly enjoy sex and let it be a celebration.

Women often struggle with relaxing control and abandoning themselves to pleasure. Some of this may be due to unfortunate double standards. The brunt of maintaining sexual control in dating relationships is placed on girls. God, in His sexual economy, makes both sexes responsible for healthy boundaries. The unhappy truth is that so often boys try to score, and girls slap hands and try to keep from getting taken advantage of, hurt, or pregnant. Wives can have a difficult time relaxing control and giving themselves permission to enjoy sexual pleasure, even in a committed and loving marital relationship.

Women also have a natural modesty that needs to be honored. They usually don't prance around naked in the locker room as men do. This is not immaturity and an inability to be "naked and unashamed" but a God-given tendency to treat bodies and sexuality with care and respect. In marriage, there is room to keep this innate modesty but also to open up to the pleasures of romping and squealing and tuning in to your child ego state, which is where great sex occurs.

## TUNING IN TO CUES

God gave each wife responsibility for her own body and for learning to experience sexual pleasure. Perhaps you are disappointed that lovemaking hasn't fallen into place as easily as you expected it to or you are not more easily orgasmic. Don't be too hard on yourself. You won't think of sex as often as your husband does, and your sexual desire will be expressed differently. You usually will have to take more time to become orgasmic, but this can be good as the sexual process is slowed down and enjoyed.

Do take control of your sexuality and tune in to cues more readily, for your own pleasure and your husband's. Here are some conscious choices that you can make (and women are much more likely to make conscious sexual choices than men) to focus in on sexual cues and keep lovemaking on the front burner of your marriage:

- Budget in and spend a certain amount of money each month on your sex life.
- Keep a mental note, and regardless of fatigue or low interest, initiate sexual activity at least once a week. You won't remember and may have to write it on the calendar.
- Have fun with your husband's visual arousal, and flaunt your nude body at unusual times just to enjoy his reactions.

- Take a bubble bath and indulge in other sensual delights at the end of a tiring day—it is a great aphrodisiac and tunes you in to your body.
- Practice Kegel exercises.

## KEGEL EXERCISES

These popular exercises are named after Dr. Arnold Kegel, who developed them in the fifties to help women with urinary incontinence. The exercises involve the pubococcygeal (PC) muscle, which connects from the pubic bone in front to the coccyx, or end of the tailbone, in back. It is one of the muscles that contracts during orgasm, increases genital awareness, and can tighten the vaginal opening. To locate this muscle, you can practice stopping the flow of urine; it can quite easily, in this fashion, be distinguished from the buttock muscles. You may feel it by inserting a finger into your vagina and trying to squeeze down on the finger.

Here are three different types of exercises that you can practice to strengthen your PC muscle. They are easy to practice while in the car, while on the telephone, or while watching television. Greater PC muscle control can increase sexual stimulation during intercourse and also help your husband's arousal.

1. Get familiar with your PC muscle as you contract and immediately relax it. Do this rapidly five times as you inhale and then exhale. Repeat five times.

2. Tighten the PC muscle for a three-second count (1001, 1002, 1003) as you inhale and then exhale and relax. Repeat ten times and then rest. Try to practice several times a day as the muscle becomes stronger.

3. Pretend your husband's penis is at the mouth of your vagina and you are trying to suck it into your vagina by pulling with your PC muscle. Pull for three seconds then relax. Repeat ten times and then rest.

## CELEBRATING UNIQUENESS

Sex therapist Debra Taylor coauthored an eye-opening book called *Secrets of Eve*, which polled two thousand Christian women. In describing what women like most about sex, physical release was fourth behind physical closeness, emotional connection, and time together. *We often have defined sexual desire through male eyes.* Frequently, a woman does not have a desire problem, but she has a fatigue problem. Or, the "problem" is simply that women do not think about sex as often as men do. Learn about yourself and celebrate that unique brand of sexual interacting that you bring to this one-flesh relationship.

## ASSERTIVE DEMANDS

You, as a woman, may enjoy a slower pace than your husband and may need different types of touching. A basic part of turning yourself on is to assertively express your needs. Sometimes you may want to cuddle and be held tight and have it lead nowhere. You may not like to always be the one to go first in having an orgasm. Now and again you may enjoy the intensity of a type of thrusting in a particular position of intercourse. Become very direct in your requests, especially in the excitement of the moment as you become a comfortable coach regarding your own needs.

The more demanding you become about your sexual needs,

the more you may turn on your husband or allow yourself to experience more pleasure. Both of you can gain skills in sexual self-awareness and assertive communication. In creating a balance that works, husbands and wives have to acknowledge and accept that their desires as to type and timing of sexual activity will not always match. Sometimes you need to say no, and at other times you will not desire to engage heavily yourself but choose to meet his sexual needs. If you stay assertive, you will keep from engaging in "duty/pity" sex, which is not fun for either partner.

## PASSIONATE POWER

You have tremendous power to arouse your husband. He desires and needs you. (A crucial note: Sometimes you won't be able to turn him on. Don't assume he's gay, having an affair, or you're not attractive. Be a detective and explore what is going on in his life. Persist through to healing and changes, even if it takes professional help.) You may be reluctant to use your feminine power, not wanting it to degenerate into destructive manipulation. But healthy and skillful sexual influencing results in a win-win situation, not the win-lose or lose-lose interaction of harmful sexual games.

Correctly using passionate power is *not* meeting him at the door in see-through lingerie so you can manipulate a designer dress out of him when you honestly cannot afford one. Healthy sexual power is not cutting off sex so he will straighten up and make needed changes. Instead, it is actively seducing your husband by playing on his visual nature so he grins all day and you delight in your femininity—or flirting and teasing in ways that increase the playfulness and fun in your sexual companionship.

## OPENLY VISUAL

Trying to be more openly visual to turn on your husband will be at first like writing with your left hand when you are right-handed. It will have to be a conscious act of will. Remember, men are aroused by seeing the female form, and the more obvious sexual parts (e.g., breasts, genitals, hips) are most powerful. Views and actions that would do nothing for you will have amazing results on your mate.

Play on his attraction to your femininity. Go upstairs in front of him and put an exaggerated swish in your hip action, knowing he is noticing and getting excited. Alone with him in his office or at home, assume a less modest sitting position— flashing him images of things to come. In lovemaking, remember to increase his visual excitement. Certain positions that are more visually stimulating, such as when you are on top, encourage his exploration and enjoyment of your genitals.

## IMMEDIATE

Your husband wants to quickly touch what he visually enjoys. Work out some appropriate compromises in which you satisfy his need for immediate gratification, but keep balance in your sex life for both your sakes. Enjoy quickies, but also teach him to postpone pleasure and not leap right to intercourse for at least five minutes. Let him nibble, but help him understand you still need to get to church in forty-five minutes. Your openness to the immediate and quick will help him back off and go more slowly.

## TEASINGLY SEDUCTIVE

Isn't it fascinating that in adolescence we are taught not to tease? Now I am telling you that teasing is a basic concept for great sex. In marriage, teasing is seductive, exhilarating, and intimate. Remember to honor your own personality and femininity as you create your own brand of seductiveness. You may never sing and dance and wear garter belts, but it is amazing how even the introvert can learn to be playful and erotic.

Tantalize him by telling him in the car on the way to dinner what you hope to do later on that night with him. The sexual tension will build during the course of the evening. While making love, your teasing comments will be met by increased arousal and excited orgasms.

## THE EXPERT LOVER

Consider the following suggestion for activities that can enhance your lovemaking. Enjoy your one-flesh companionship. Men, though predictable, are not always easy to live with sexually. They are wired in some seemingly crazy ways, but you can enjoy your sexual power with your husband.

### FOCUSING ON YOUR HUSBAND'S BODY

Because men are usually more easily stimulated physically and visually, couples neglect to focus attention and energy on the husband's body. Your husband may feel uncomfortable at first, but throughout the loveplay, keep your hands on him. It should not be a focus on his genital area. Hold and caress and stroke his body. You will probably find he ejaculates less quickly as you touch and hold more.

Don't let your husband get away with focusing only on your body! Sensually massage, and help him learn to enjoy back rubs and facials. Practice two-minute embraces. Don't neglect caressing during intercourse. Holding his testicles gently or massaging the prostate or reaching down and placing your index and middle finger like scissors at the mouth of your vagina to grasp his penis going in and out can all bring extra delight. Assertively insist on nurturing him physically. Like so many things in life, as he tries it, he will like it.

## SPECIAL STIMULATION

Making love to your husband's penis is crucial to turning him on. The penis is a part of your husband's anatomy that he is proud and protective of, but it is not fragile. Intimacy is his entrusting you with this very personal part of himself. Rapid and firm strokes are usually more stimulating. Develop a rhythm and pressure that he enjoys.

Orally stimulating the penis is very exciting for most men. In oral sex, probably your mouth and lips are not strong enough to give sufficient stimulation for building toward an orgasm. The fun is more in the teasing and the intimacy of his entrusting his penis to your mouth rather than just creating orgasms. Manually stroking the shaft while focusing on the head of the penis with your mouth can bring real enjoyment. Greater sensation exists in the head of the penis. Shield your teeth with your lips pulled over them as you orally stimulate with tongue, lips, and mouth. If you don't want him to climax in your mouth, he has control—just tell him.

In intercourse, practice your Kegel exercises with your mate's penis in your vagina. That can be arousing for both of you. Allow him to feel your PC muscle enclose and tighten on his penis. Have him do this with just the head of the penis as he gently thrusts into the mouth of your vagina and you tighten the PC muscle. Play and experiment—sex is fun.

## SEXUAL FLOODING

Many husbands dream about being ravished by so much sex they couldn't stand more. At a time when you are feeling relaxed and rested—it may have to be on vacation—tell your mate that he is free to initiate sex whenever he desires and that you will be disappointed if it is not very frequent. Quickies will be fine as well as long, drawn-out lovemaking.

Help him out by planning some sexual sessions that appeal to his specific visual orientation. Place him on the bed, or wherever, and let him get aroused with some anticipation as you get your props (lingerie, music, etc.) ready. Then overwhelm him with sexy apparel, sexy movements, and sexy sights of your body clothed and nude. Plan exciting surprises of your own during this time. Create a flood of sexual activity.

## POWER POSITIONS

Be sure to read the chapter on creative positions for intercourse. While enjoying intercourse, remember your husband's penchant for looking and touching. Learn to flaunt your body as you exercise your power to turn him on. Encourage him to caress and explore. It is an intensely sensuous experience for him to run his penis or a finger over your clitoris, gently down to your vagina, and slowly into it—the warmth and moistness and unique femininity are very arousing. You have tremendous power with your femininity—exercise it during intercourse. Most women, as they get comfortable with their capacity to be seductive, find themselves aroused by this ability.

May you have courage, spontaneity, zest, love, and a whole lot of fun as you turn your man on. The rewards of learning new skills are great. Take a walk on the male side of life. You will find yourself enjoying your sexuality a lot more and your relationship reaching new depths.

## TIME OUT . . .

With a female friend, discuss the messages you have incorporated into your sex life and where they came from. Look at your father and mother's attitudes on sex, your childhood, your high school years and your first sexual experiences, any traumas, and your marriage. Which attitude(s) will you choose to alter? Discuss with her the concept of female power, how your desire is real but different from your husband's, and the difference between nurturing sex and duty sex.

*10*

# THE HONEYMOON

*T*he word *honeymoon* conjures up feelings of exciting adventures, sexual beginnings, and playful vacationing. It can live up to this and more, but like a great sex life, a fantastic honeymoon doesn't just happen. Quite often couples come into my counseling office with problems that go back to these beginning experiences.

If you have already read the book up to this point, you probably have knowledge and skills that will help you head off many of the common honeymoon pitfalls. This chapter can help you further in getting rid of some unrealistic expectations, do some needed strategic planning, and be prepared for possible challenges as you pull off a memorable time of playful sex and intimate bonding.

In writing this chapter I polled the many couples in the newlyweds class that I teach and interviewed all my friends, inquiring what I should include in this chapter. These answers and my years of listening to stories have produced four crucial areas to focus on: the honeymoon objectives, the wedding night, possible challenges, and honeymooning through the first two years.

## HONEYMOON OBJECTIVES

One couple told me to warn honeymooners not to tour England in ten days in November. They felt they could write the "How Not To" book. We laughed, but this is a great place to start in thinking through what are the ingredients and goals of a great honeymoon.

*Rest and relaxation.* You will be exhausted after the wedding and the months leading up to it. A wise marriage mentor asked me to encourage couples to take two weeks for their honeymoon. She knew it would be expensive but saw a huge importance in rest and this initial time together. She thought that the two weeks should become a financial objective within the wedding plans. This time truly helps you recuperate from the wedding, bond with each other, and prepare for the coming stressful months.

*Privacy and time alone.* Your marriage is new, and you are infatuated with this novel experience and with each other. You two could feel alone and connected even in a crowd, but private time is still important. Some settings are much more conducive to this. If you go to Disneyland, allow some fun hotel time too. Gaze deeply into your lover's eyes, keep your hands on intimate zones, and drink each other up—preferably not in public places.

*Great sex.* The first nine chapters will help with needed skills and attitudes. Relax and plan in a lot of playtime. One friend, who was a virgin when he married, told me that on his honeymoon he wanted to do everything he had chosen not to do for the past fifteen years. He related that it may not have been like the movies, but they took showers together, romped naked, and had great fun making whoopee.

Take a break from sex once in a while and enjoy an exercise called *sensate focus*. One partner will be the passive receiver and the other will be the active giver for fifteen minutes—then exchange roles. Both partners should be nude for this experience and increase sensuality with a pleasant lotion. If you are the active giver, touch and caress your mate in ways that bring pleasure to you. There is no right way to do this because you are touching for your own pleasure. If your mate does not like to be touched in certain areas, refrain out of love and respect. The passive partner will enjoy receiving pleasurable massage and pleasing you. The passive receiver is learning what touch feels best personally and what kind of active touch you like to give. This exercise focuses on Level Three and Level Two erogenous zones (see Chapter 2). There should be no touching of the genital area and nipples. Do not go on to making love during these sessions.

*Planned activities and recreation.* You need time to rest and have sex, but recreational activity is very bonding too. Tailor your honeymoon to each of your personalities and preferences. Most likely one of you is active and one can veg more easily. You are starting habits and creating rituals for a lifetime. Plan in some memorable moments. You may prefer a beach resort or Disneyland or something like a cruise where someone else has done the planning and you can choose to participate or not. Remember to think through some of the little things that can become a nuisance, such as where you will eat.

*Reasonable financial objectives.* Knowing you are coming back to unreasonable debt can be a real downer. Make sure to plan your honeymoon into the wedding budget. Two extra days may be more important than nicer flowers. You are reinforcing your future financial habits. Don't be a tightwad. You are recreating and making memories. At the same time be smart—a new couch will last much longer than that sailboat ride.

Be sure to sit down together and discuss the above objectives and any others that may seem important to you. The place, activities, and setting must fit in with your objectives and personal styles. You are trying to *plan through a memorable time* as you eliminate as many *unpleasant surprises* and *disappointed expectations* as you can.

## THE WEDDING NIGHT

Let me share with you some wise advice I have gleaned over the years about the wedding night. Here is one comment that gives perspective: "This is the first of twenty-five thousand nights. Relax, talk, and keep your sense of humor." Take the time to discuss each of the following ideas as you plan and sort through that first twelve hours as man and wife. Please take away the spirit of these suggestions.

Sex therapist and friend Christopher McCluskey tells how his father advised him not to push for intercourse on the wedding night. He encouraged them to relax, perhaps take a warm bath together, and begin the process of knowing each other as mates. Chris relates what wise advice this was and the pressures that were removed as he followed it. Taking the opportunity to connect emotionally and spiritually before the physical consummation created a greater feeling of safety and intimacy with each other.

A colleague, known for his organization and business skills, passionately stated, "I hope they don't let this night just happen.

I don't care how much they love spontaneity or how busy they are, trust me—this twenty-four hours needs planning." He went on to explain how their planning and discussion ahead of time really helped pave the way for a great night and the whole next day. They were exhausted and traveled only twenty minutes from the reception to the hotel and paid for two nights, staying until late the next afternoon. He hastened to add that he didn't plan everything out and there was much spontaneous play and laughter, but the planning was important.

A pastor pleaded, "Just because they have already had sex, don't let them treat their wedding night in an ordinary way. This is their first time of truly making love. Let them build on their new covenant as they discover exciting and deeper levels of sexual intimacy." Plan surprises and luxuriate in the intimacy of this honeymoon connecting time. Read through Chapters 8 and 9 again. Go beyond your bachelor's degree in each other. Start to work on your Ph.D. in your mate and the true art of making love. There are levels of commitment and touching each other's bodies and hearts that you haven't achieved but need to incorporate into your new love life. Make this a special time as you begin this journey as husband and wife.

A marriage and family therapist wanted to emphasize, "The first twelve hours are setting patterns for the future intimacy of their marriage. They need to let God's warm love and gentle wisdom permeate their relationship." Be sensitive and empathetic to what each of you needs. You are learning to communicate about private and core issues. Be patient, not critical. I remember the client who spoke with pain in her voice about her husband's chance comment on their first intercourse: "He told me that he thought I should move more." She was trying so hard in her inexperience, and this little criticism wounded her deeply. Gently talk and support each other as you patiently understand and lovingly empathize.

If you are virgins, what can help that first experience be exciting? Women, it is important to get a gynecological exam before the honeymoon. This can help to determine if the hymen or vagina is tight or identify other possible difficulties such as vaginal scar tissue or infections. Take time to relax and begin getting comfortable with each other. One mom had the foresight to tell her daughter, "Remember, he will want to see you naked." With her natural female modesty, she was apprehensive but more prepared.

A shower, kissing, and caressing with mutual genital exploration and explanation can begin the "knowing" process. One friend told me that what helped him the most was constant communication and the ability to laugh together. Relax before attempting intercourse and get in a comfortable position. Keep communicating and allow the wife to give permission to enter and to guide the process. Use some lubrication and go slowly with inserting the penis. If it feels like there is no vaginal opening, she may be tight or you may not have spread the labia open enough. The pain of breaking the hymen varies, with some women feeling only mild discomfort. If the pain gets too intense, wait and try again later. Keep talking as you laugh and learn together.

## POSSIBLE CHALLENGES

Every wedding and honeymoon has glitches and mishaps. There are things you couldn't plan for and things you have to learn together. How you handle these challenges can make a huge difference in your future marriage and sex life. Here are common challenges with some suggestions.

*The environment disappoints.* One couple related how they went to Bermuda and drank the water. Diarrhea and vomiting were almost too much intimacy for a beginning marriage. Another couple who planned for two weeks alone ended up with honeymoon cystitis. Others have reported that despite planning, the wife started her period on the day of the wedding. Keep your sense of humor and know there are many more years for sex. You are still creating fun memories. Have a wise mentor, probably not your parents, picked out to call if things really get depressed or crazy and you need quick advice or support.

*A lack of knowledge strikes.* I quote from a recently married couple: "I did not realize how hard it would be to figure out the act of making love. Every guy has heard the myth of sixteen times on the wedding night. Counter to popular opinion, sex does not work like clockwork; it is more similar to putting a jigsaw puzzle together with several pieces missing." Reading this book will help, but there is no substitute for practice. Give each other permission to be naive, and courageously begin to work through your skill deficits.

*Anxiety reigns.* Anxiousness can hinder erection, create premature ejaculation, lessen vaginal lubrication, and interrupt playfulness. Awkwardness is normal, but crippling performance anxiety can be lessened with some preplanning. The husband can be reassured that he doesn't have to know all about sex. He may have come into the marriage feeling very incompetent. Know that all problems can be worked through with help.

Keep playing and enjoying each other as you work through the sexual barriers to solutions.

*Repression hurts.* You have so carefully guarded your sexuality and set such rigid boundaries that you have repressed your sexual feelings. Your wedding vows are not the switch that will turn these back on. Nudity and sexual activity may be scary or even repulsive at first. God has given you the feelings, and He will help you achieve the wonderful lovemaking that you long for. Be patient with yourself and each other as you turn your sexual rheostat from very dim to bright. This will indeed take time.

*Desire disappears.* A lack of sexual desire is a very complex issue and can show up on the honeymoon. You can think through common causes like abuse or repression, but this will most likely need some professional help. Dating may have been controlled enough to engage in passionate kissing but making love may prove to be too much. Enjoy physical affection and get help when you get back home to sort through needed changes.

*Guilt and mistakes haunt.* You are not a virgin and you have herpes. Hopefully, this has been talked through before the honeymoon. Forgiveness and acceptance can take time, and the honeymoon can trigger the guilt. Pray together for healing and the wisdom to overcome the consequences of sin as you appropriate deeper forgiveness before and during the honeymoon.

*Brokenness invades.* One out of three women have had a sexually traumatizing experience by the time they are seventeen, and the statistics on men are very similar. For some, the trauma of these experiences may begin to interfere with sexual response on the honeymoon. If this happens, try to stay in the present moment of lovemaking. Gently but assertively stop as needed. The unwounded mate must be patient and gain understanding. You are healing agents for each other and will work through this over time with professional help.

*Physical pain persists.* You may have had a medical exam, but this will not always deter all problems. After the honeymoon you may need a second opinion. It may also be anxiety and a need for extra lubrication or going slow. Pain obviously has a dampening effect on sexual pleasure. Sometimes with tightness of the vagina or the breaking of the hymen, pain can diminish over the honeymoon, but a good rule of thumb is not to play through real sexual pain. Stop as needed and get help if the pain persists.

*The husband misfires.* Premature ejaculation because of excitement is common, especially in young men. Masters and Johnson state that with active thrusting, most men climax in under two minutes. The amount of sex on the honeymoon will help him last longer, but there are exercises to help prolong intercourse. Do some reading and get help in your first year.

*The wife takes time.* A couple shared how disappointed and frustrated they were that it took them three months of experimenting and learning before she became orgasmic. This is not unusual, and becoming orgasmic should not be the focus of the honeymoon. Unlike men, women typically can take fifteen to thirty minutes of direct stimulation to reach an orgasm. This can be even longer when she is just learning her sexual responsiveness.

*A crash course on understanding differences occurs.* He wants to hike and she wants to romantically sun together on the beach. She comes into the bathroom uninvited. He wants to eat in bed. Welcome to marriage. But the honeymoon is not an ideal time to feel relational pain and to be angry with each other. That is why a helpful course in communication and conflict resolution and some effective premarital counseling can greatly help these first weeks and months as partners.

With all of these challenges, have the wisdom to not let them become destructive strongholds in your marriage in the coming months and years. Assertively talk them through and seek professional help early if needed.

## HONEYMOONING THE FIRST TWO YEARS

The honeymoon begins the fun journey of becoming lovers and partners. Remember that it is the beginning and the goals will not all be accomplished in one or two weeks. It is vital to continue the playing and transitions and problem solving in the next year or two. "When a man has taken a new wife, he shall not go out to war or be charged with any business; he shall be free at home one year, and bring happiness to his wife" (Deut. 24:5). Here are some of my encouragements:

*Work through the challenges.* Don't let them become barriers as you nondefensively seek out the needed help. She may need to check out the pain and perhaps stretch her vagina over the coming months as she reduces anxiety and pain. That sexual abuse may finally have to be faced. A sex therapist can help with the premature ejaculation or desire issues. Your stress reduction may involve learning better communication skills or finding a financial planner.

*Become orgasmic.* It is not unusual that wives have not explored themselves and already experienced an orgasm. What does a female orgasm feel like? If you wonder if you have had an orgasm, you probably haven't. Buy my book *A Celebration of Sex* and work through the exercises together. Be patient but persistent.

*Create greater sexual intimacy.* Read more and make the time for playing at sex. It can help to read out loud to each other from a sexual book. Start with this one. Set aside date nights and gourmet sex nights where you play for hours. Try new positions and get some props to accent sensuality.

*Build your marriage skills.* Go to some workshops. There are many great books on marriage; read one together. Find some other couples with solid marriages and hang out with them. Join a community group. Get some more training in building better conflict resolution skills or financial management. A great marriage creates great sex.

*Make extra time for each other.* The first two years should have more vacations and times to retreat into the privacy of your home and bedroom. You are creating a lifetime partnership, and hours of communicating will be necessary. Consider these years sabbatical years in which you say no to other obligations and yes to each other.

Thanks for reading this book. I'm proud of you. A great marriage and a fantastic sex life are marvelous testimonies to the Creator's intimate love. May God bless and guide your ongoing journey into His awesome world of intimacy.

# ACKNOWLEDGMENTS

*C*atherine Rosenau, my admired and appreciated companion, has once again supported me through another book. Thank you for being my lover and soul mate.

My special friends and fellow sex therapists in Sexual Wholeness, Inc. (Christopher McCluskey, Debra Taylor, Michael Sytsma) have helped shape this book and my life. Thanks so much for your support and love.

A special thanks for the helpful input of my current class of engaged and newlyweds at North Point Community Church and my co-teachers, Scott and Amy Reed. Over many years I have learned so much about newlyweds in teaching this class.

Appreciation is given to my illustrator, Alan Tiegreen, who created the drawings and helped me rework some for this book.

Elizabeth Kea at Thomas Nelson helped make many wise and skillful decisions in creating this book as she worked her editorial magic with tremendous talent.

Thank you, Victor Oliver, for taking a chance many years ago on an unknown author and working to get books on sexuality published.

# About the Author

Douglas Rosenau, Ed.D., is a licensed psychologist, marriage and family therapist, and diplomate of the American Board of Sexology (ABS). A pioneer in Christian sex therapy, Dr. Rosenau is the bestselling author of *A Celebration of Sex* and has written numerous articles on healthy sexuality for such publications as *Christian Counseling Today* and *New Man*. He is a full clinical member of the Society for Sex Therapy and Research (SSTAR) and teaches human sexuality as an adjunct professor at Reformed Theological Seminary and Psychological Studies Institute. As cofounder of the Christian organization Sexual Wholeness, Doug has helped to create the Institute for Sexual Wholeness, a cooperative venture with the Psychological Studies Institute, which trains Christian sex therapists, creates teaching videos and materials, and encourages research.

Dr. Rosenau and his wife, Cathy, live in Atlanta, Georgia, and have a daughter, Merrill, son-in-law, Tom, and granddaughter, Caitlyn, who is the apple of his eye.

If you would like more information on Dr. Rosenau's resources and seminars, contact:

Sexual Wholeness, Inc.
P.O. Box 550911
Atlanta, GA 30355-3411
phone: (404) 705-7077
www.sexualwholeness.com